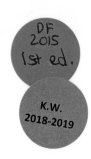
10200

humor
and the health
professions

vera m. robinson

Library of Congress catalog card number: 77-777-92

Printed in the United States of America by

[C][B][S]   Charles B. Slack, Inc.
6900 Grove Road
Thorofare, N.J. 08086

preface

Humor is a form of communication highly regarded in our society. As the vast amount of literature can attest, there has always been a need for laughter and comedy. Humor has been described as a pleasure upon which man pounces at the slightest excuse for indulging in it. No one denies its value. It is a part of our lives even in times of stress, danger, and death. Yet, despite our recognition of its value, we do not take humor seriously. Somehow, we are afraid to look at it, to analyze it, and to make conscious, deliberate use of humor as a tool in communication, as a way of intervening in the stresses of living. We allow it to happen by chance. Particularly in the health professions, there is generally no attempt at a planned use of humor.

The time is ripe for health professionals to do more than just enjoy humor. We need to understand it. We need to begin to be able to laugh at ourselves, at life, and at our establishments. We need to begin to help our students and patients to deal with their stresses, tensions and frustrations through the use of humor. We need to believe that humor is constructive and healthy; we must encourage its use as a coping mechanism, and cultivate its use as a viable tool in communication. ⸺

The aim of this study is to go beyond the description and theorizing about the nature of humor — which has been the primary focus of other authors and researchers — to providing some beginning guidelines for cultivating this concept of humor as a planned tool in teaching, in communication, and in intervention.

In order to accomplish this purpose, a foundation of understanding regarding the nature of humor is a logical first step. An overview of the varied and conflicting theories, the issues, controversies, and past studies will form the first part of this book.

Section II takes a look at the current utilization of humor in health settings and by the helping professionals. What purpose does it serve? How does it fit into the usual pattern of communication? How does "medical" humor (between staff) differ from humor used with patients or clients? How has humor been used in the teaching-learning process? How has humor been used in mental health, in psychotherapy as a therapeutic tool?

If one is, then, to make conscious use of humor, what variables would need to be considered if the attempt is to be constructive and successful? Does everyone have a "sense of humor?" How is it acquired? Is one "born" with a sense of humor or is it "developed?" Does age make a difference in appreciation of humor? Do the personalities of the individuals involved make a difference? Does the culture of the patient make a difference?

Finally, although much more investigation and research needs to be conducted, some beginning guidelines for cultivating the use of humor are suggested. Elements of comedy and techniques for producing comedy are gleaned from the works of comedy writers and comedians, and developed as a guide for creating humor. There are suggestions for incorporating humor in the teaching-learning process as a means for facilitating learning and as a model for students, as well as suggestions for teaching the concept of humor and the utilization of humor as a tool in intervention in the helping process.

The belief that humor is necessary to human welfare and as a survival mechanism to cope with the "heavies of living" is shared by many. In the enthusiasm and urging that we not lose this great benefit, we may end up appearing to propose a "prescription" or "recipe," which may seem too mechanical. Actually, these "prescriptions" are the plant food and fertilizer to aid in the growth of humor. The key word to remember is *cultivate*. We can teach, or facilitate the learning of, the knowledge about, the concept of humor, but the attitude, the "sense of humor," must be enculturated. Cultivation implies the right atmosphere, patience, and loving care, with the occasional application of artificial aids for revitalization and stimulation.

A companion concept which has been suggested is that of "habituation." The cultivation of humor requires consistent exposure and practice. Together with the understanding of the concept of humor, the "sense of humor" comes into bloom.

He who laughs, lasts.
ANON

acknowledgments

Although my interest in humor goes way back, my first research in this area originated with a Western Council for Higher Education in Nursing project in which representatives from 24 schools of nursing met to develop mental health concepts for integrating into nursing curricula. That group collected anecdotes, shared their humor, and reviewed initial drafts of my first study. I would like to acknowledge their support. Appreciation is due to Marguerite Cobb who critiqued my work midway in the project and first encouraged me to write a book. I would also like to thank Thelma M. Schorr who provided editorial consultation on the final draft and dared us to have some original thoughts! That material became Chapter 7 of *Behavioral Concepts and Nursing Intervention* published by J.B. Lippincott in 1970.

I would also like to acknowledge the enthusiastic support and participation from 1965-1970, during that initial study, of the faculty of the School of Nursing of the University of Northern Colorado, the staff of Weld County General Hospital and the nursing students who lived through our humorous attempts.

My continuing research in the ensuing years in the area of humor during my doctoral study which culminated in this book was achieved through the innovative School of Educational Change and Development at the University of Northern Colorado.

I would like to extend a very special thank-you to Dr. Donald G. Decker, first Dean of the School of Educational Change and Development, for his initial encouragement and warm support, and to Dr. Donald M. Luketich, present Dean, who continued that support.

To my Resource Board, I will always be indebted. Their careful and provocative thought, their guidance, encouragement, and good humor supported me throughout my doctoral studies and in the writing of this book. Dr. Franklin D. Cordell supervised my progress and guided the development of the research projects. Dr. John W. Harrison steadfastly and diligently reviewed and critiqued each chapter and provided guidance and references in the area of Black Humor and other comedy references. Dr. Lola J. Montgomery supervised the area of personality and the sense of humor.

To my four Consultants, Dr. Barbara H. Mickey, Dr. Eunice M. Blair, Dean Elaine M. Mengis and Assistant Dean Elda S. Popiel who also gave of their time and expertise in special areas, I am most grateful. Dr. Mickey first suggested a narrowing of the research and guided the development of the chapter on culture.

I would also like to thank the faculty and students at the University of Colorado and all the many colleagues in the community agencies who participated in the two studies in this book. Specifically, I would like to thank Pat Meecham, Nancy Zalewski, Joanne Ruth, and Bobbie Taylor who shared their studies as graduate students; Virginia Carozza, Sophronia Williams, Jessie Baus, Lydia Pourier, and Mary Drake who shared their thoughts and experiences in the development of the chapter on culture; Patsy Perry, Maureen Rausch, Margaret Ball, Carole Anderson, Gwen Stephens, and Margaret Williams whose comments and humorous examples in teaching I have used; and Signe Cooper and Mary F. Hill whose humor I have related. To all the other many, many colleagues, friends, students and patients over the years who provided me with jokes, references, and examples of humor, who participated in my studies, who reacted to my writing, laughed at my jokes, and encouraged me, I would like to express my heartfelt appreciation. I wish I could name them all, but that would be another book in itself.

Of course, no acknowledgment would be complete without recognizing the efforts of my secretarial assistants who typed, proofread, and copied the many drafts of the manuscript: Joan Hamilton, Betty Jean Brown, Marjorie Frandsen, and Mary Regan.

Finally, but not least, I wish to acknowledge my family: husband, Frank; daughters, Elizabeth and Elaine; son, Bill; and my mother, without whose love, support, prodding and jokes, I would never have made it to this point of completion.

introduction

*To everything there is a season, and a
time to every purpose under the heaven:
a time to weep, and a time to laugh; a
time to mourn, and a time to dance.*

ECCLESIASTES 3:4

The past two decades have seen an increasing emphasis within the helping professions on a more humanistic approach to the individual. We recognize each person as a psychosocial being with his own unique perceptions, motivations, and behaviors. In times of illness and stress, we focus on relating to the patient as a human being, not just a biological organism. We accept him as he is and where he is, with all his problems, weaknesses, and deficiencies, as well as his strengths. We accept him as a person worthy of our respect, our caring, and our understanding. Essentially, we accept his humanness, that is, not only his potential for success, but his potential for failure, his potential for tragedy, and his potential for comedy.

Within this humanistic framework of openness and warmth, humor is a natural phenomenon. As man's self-concept develops, as he becomes more tolerant and more understanding of himself and of others, the more he is able to laugh at himself and at his imperfections, and to share this common bond with others.

In the helping professions we have analyzed many of the behaviors of man: anxiety, frustration, conflict, aggression. We have recognized man's need to cry and to grieve and have investigated the grieving process extensively. We have not, however, given the same degree of attention to grief's counterpart: man's need to laugh!

Yet humor is as common a behavior as all the others. In fact, humor is a way of life in our society. It permeates every aspect of our existence. Observe any group, in any setting, at home, at work, at play, in the street, the office, the factory, the prison, the sick room, even the funeral home, and you will hear laughter and humorous interchange. The humor may range from a smile and a simple pleasantry to a joke-telling, slapstick session, but it is there.

In almost any book concerning human behavior one finds references to the benefits of humor. In every list of admirable characteristics of human behavior, a sense of humor always appears. Yet no one indicates how this great benefit or important behavior should be capitalized upon — how it should be cultivated. It is simply allowed to happen or not.

> Our sense of humor is, without a doubt, one of our most valuable faculties.... Yet no one seems to know how to cultivate their own, or anybody else's, sense of humor.[1]

Perhaps, because humor is such a pervasive element in our lives and one which we enjoy and anticipate rather than dread or avoid, we fail to take it seriously or to evaluate it in regard to its benefits, its effects or the cues it gives us to the individual for whom we are caring. Certainly, in the health professions, we have made little planned use of the concept of humor in communication, as a mechanism for coping with stress, or as a catalyst in the teaching-learning process.

To say that humor should be taken seriously is a paradox in itself; yet once we pass through the analytic stage, so that we understand humor, should we not be able, as with any other concept, to be more spontaneous and actually appreciate humor more? To paraphrase: Humor is not just a laughing matter, it is a serious business!

Martin Grotjahn contends that "he who understands the comic begins to understand humanity and the struggle for freedom and happiness."[2] He expresses the hope "that we may laugh even more merrily and with greater inner freedom when we understand laughter better."

This book is a beginning effort in this direction: to pull together the vast amount of literature into a body of knowledge, make application to its use in health care settings, and suggest beginning guidelines for cultivating the use of humor in our interactions and interventions with our patients and clients.

REFERENCES

1. Mindess H: *Laughter and Liberation.* Los Angeles, Nash Publishing Co, 1971, p 13.
2. Grotjahn M: *Beyond Laughter.* New York, Blakiston Division, McGraw-Hill Book Co, 1957, pp VII-IX.

table of contents

1 the nature of humor

2 humor in health and illness

3 cultivating the use of humor

1 the nature of humor

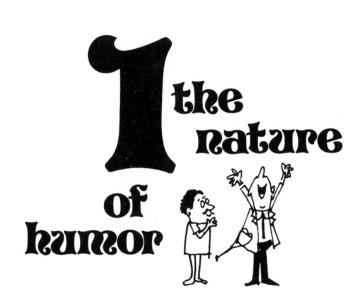

paradoxes, 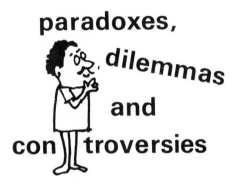 dilemmas and con troversies

What is humor? What is the nature of humor? What is it that makes us laugh? Why does man need to laugh? These are questions that men have pondered for centuries.

> Comedy...has been one of mankind's persistent modes of thought, of action, of self-awareness. Men have always written comedies; they have, as well, tried to explain why. No single satisfactory answer has emerged.[1]

The concept of humor has been considered and discussed by man as far back in time as he could express himself in writing and probably long before that. Humor has been discussed from the point of view of philosophers, psychologists, psychoanalysts, anthropologists, sociologists, physiologists, dramatists, playwrights, poets, prose writers, satirists, comedians, educators, child development specialists, industrial management specialists *ad infinitum.* No area of human behavior or endeavor apparently has neglected the concept of humor.

Man has attempted to define and categorize humor, to describe its nature, its causes, its effects, its purposes, and usefulness, to analyze the elements which produce it, and, of course, to create it.

As a matter of fact, so much has been written and speculated that each new author or theorist feels impelled to review all the past literature and thoughts before he attempts his own. Somehow, the same unique pattern occurs: the author first apologizes for the complexities involved in discussing this subject and then proceeds to present each of the past theories or writings in turn. Each theory appears to have a quality of reasonableness and validity but, as the reader is nodding his head in agreement, the author promptly tears that theory apart and proves its inadequacy. By the time the author arrives at his own theory, which he says is an attempt to bring some order out of the chaos and provide a better explanation of the nature of humor, the reader is exhausted and thoroughly confused!

The situation becomes so ludicrous that one wonders if this is not a joke on humanity by Nature, who is holding her sides in helpless laughter at man's ludicrous attempt to analyze that phenomenon he has defined in terms of the ludicrous!

It has the quality of a Robert Frost:

> "Forgive, Oh Lord, my little jokes on thee, and I'll forgive
> thy great big one on me."[2]

However, to the reader, it soon becomes apparent that the difficulty lies in the fact that each has been attempting to find a single all-inclusive answer, when actually there seems to be no one answer to the nature and purpose of humor. It is a combination of many factors and it serves many purposes; and the nature and purpose will vary depending upon the situation. There are still many unanswered questions about the concept of humor, and there is still much controversy and a lack of consensus.

One of the biggest dilemmas in this area of humor is caused by the very fact that there is no universally accepted language or theoretical framework for this concept. Essentially it cuts across so many disciplines and areas of study that it belongs nowhere and yet everywhere. Each discipline ends up defining humor from its own perspective, which is never complete in itself.

Perhaps the very nature of humor creates the difficulties we find in analyzing, studying, collecting data and attempting to develop theories.

Humor has been very aptly described as a paradox. To be effective, humor requires a spontaneity, an element of surprise. There is a spontaneity-thoughtfulness balance. If we become too thoughtful or too self-conscious about it, we lose it! Once we stop to analyze a joke, it is no longer funny! Have you ever tried to explain a joke to someone who did not "get it?"

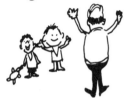

> Humor can be dissected, as a frog can, but the thing dies in the process and the innards are discouraging to any but the pure scientific mind.[3]

Play also requires this same spontaneity-thoughtfulness balance, and humor is considered within the framework of play. Both are imbued with a feeling of enjoyment, fantasy, and freedom because of the element of unreality. This is "not real," it is "just fun," it is "just a joke." Both are looked on as "trivial"; yet both function within very definite rules and a serious undertone. Humor is the only form of play usually acceptable in a predominantly serious situation.

> Behind the smoke screen of the official definition of humor as trivial, humor functions as a mode of indirect communication in the most serious of matters.[4]

There is almost no situation in life — not even dying — about which humor is not possible. Yet the responsibility associated with the seriousness is absolved in humor.

One can retreat with, "I was just joking. I didn't really mean it."

Another paradox in the concept of humor is created by its subjective quality. Humor can be very individual in that what is very funny to one person may not be funny at all to another!

Not only is this a result of the individual's own uniqueness, but humor also is situational. Humor flows out of the interaction within a particular setting or situation, and to appreciate that humorous incident requires a knowledge of the culture or situation. There may be a need for a knowledge base or necessary background information. The persons involved may react with hilarity, but an outsider may wonder, "What was so funny?"

In a lecture on brain tumors, a nursing instructor was discussing the methods for pinpointing the location of the tumor and the importance of doing so prior to surgery. She said "You can grub around in an abdomen, but you can't grub around in a brain!" The student nurses roared with laughter. To the lay person, who did not understand the anatomy and physiology involved and the ludicrousness of "grubbing" in the brain, this comment might even be repugnant, let alone unfunny.

These paradoxes create problems in attempts to observe and study humor or collect data in natural settings. Empirical studies to validate theoretical constructs about humor are often questioned because there are not enough data from natural settings to provide a norm against which studies can be judged.

In direct observation of any communication we know that the presence of another person affects that interaction. When humor is known to be the topic of observation, one of two reactions occur. Either the person or group becomes so self-conscious that the humor disappears, or quite the opposite occurs (which is another paradox), the quantity of humor increases. People try harder to be funny! Humor is contagious! One joking comment leads to another!

Joan Emerson, in a doctoral study in 1962 investigating the social functions of humor in a hospital setting, spent eight months collecting data. She stated:

> To observe relatively unself-conscious interaction it was
> necessary to stay in one setting long enough to accustom
> the subjects to the presence of the observer.[4]

She sat in on the course given to Nurse's Aides and often participated in the ongoing activity while observing the interactions of the staff with the patients. She had to be available and as unobtrusive a part of the normal routine as possible in order to be there when the humor occurred. And yet, her observer's role was often regarded as a joking matter and her following the subjects around provoked humor.

The other approach to collecting data in natural settings is to ask the individuals within the settings to record their own humorous interactions. This poses another problem. Since humor is spontaneous and more often situational, the individual gets "caught up" in the exchange and forgets to record. Later, when one tries to recall the incident, it is often difficult to remember the details, unless it was exceptionally funny. Or this kind of humorous interaction was such an integral component of the communication pattern that the participant does not relate to the fact of humor, or does not consider it a humorous incident. Often, the person will say, "They laughed, but I don't know what I did that was so funny!"

Humor becomes such an integral part of the ongoing life processes that recording its occurrences forces one to an unnatural degree of self-consciousness. The self-consciousness, then, operates to create a different mood, and the humor has gone.[5]

As a result, despite the initial enthusiasm by the participants in collecting data for the researcher, the results are often meager.

The researcher, also, in reading the observations has difficulty seeing "what was funny" because he was not in the situation.

Because collecting original data in natural settings becomes a long and difficult process, others have attempted to control the situations by experimental studies in the laboratory. This obviously creates problems in terms of the spontaneity and raises the question of salience: that is, whatever happens to be the salient topic is the one that arouses the humor.

However, it is obvious that much more research into humor and into methods for investigation of humor must be done. Despite all of the barriers, the studies do go on. Humor is a phenomenon which continues to intrigue man.

REFERENCES

1. Felheim M (ed): *Comedy: Plays, Theory, and Criticism.* New York, Harcourt, Brace and World, 1962, p V.
2. Frost R: Forgive, O Lord. *In the Clearing.* New York, Holt, Rinehart and Winston, 1962, p 39.
3. White EB: Some Remarks on Humor. *In* Enck JJ, Forter, ET, Whitley, A (eds): *The Comic in Theory and Practice.* New York, Appleton-Century-Crofts, 1960, p 102.
4. Emerson JP: *Social Functions of Humor in a Hospital Setting.* Unpublished dissertation, University of California, Berkeley, 1963, p 10.
5. *Ibid,* p 4.
6. Fry WF Jr: *Sweet Madness.* Palo Alto, California, Pacific Books, 1963, p 5.

def-i-ni-tions of humor

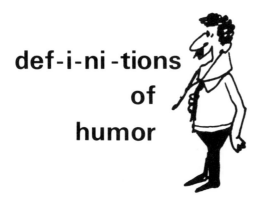

Finding a universal definition for humor is as difficult as finding a universal language or theory. Many authors simply avoid the issue by not defining it!

Webster defines humor as "that quality which appeals to a sense of the ludicrous or absurdly incongruous" and lists the archaic definition of humor *(umor)* as *moisture, vapor.*

In old medieval physiology, *humor* referred to the four principal fluids of the body: blood, phlegm, cholor (yellow bile), and melancholy (black bile). The predominance of any of these fluids determined man's health or temperament or mood. A just balance made a good compound called "good humor," and a preponderance of any one made a bad compound called "ill humor." We still speak of a person's "good humor."

Others have defined humor from their own particular perspectives. Crothers called humor *the frank enjoyment of the imperfect.* Stephen Leacock defined it as the *kindly contemplation of the incongruities of life and the artistic contemplation thereof.*

Many define humor operationally in relation to laughter and describe laughter as the indicator that humor has occurred. The two terms are often used interchangeably. However, other behavioral responses are also considered indications of amusement: that is, smiling, change in facial expression, twinkling eyes, etc.

To complicate the situation, there are a myriad of other related terms, which many have attempted to distinguish, such as wit, satire, punning, clowning, teasing, joking, comedy, practical joking, pantomine, sarcasm, cartoons, etc.

So as not to be snared in the trap of attempting all these distinctions, a more generic definition usually provides for the breadth and varieties of humor which can occur in a natural setting. Since humor is being viewed as a medium of communication in health settings, it will be more useful to define humor as any communication which is perceived by any of the interacting parties as humorous and leads to laughing, smiling, or a feeling of amusement.

Most of the humor within health settings is spontaneous or situational in nature rather than of the formal joke-telling or practical joke variety. Formal humor may be literary works, planned inclusions of jokes, cartoons or funny stories in speeches, lectures, TV shows, or other formal situations. Spontaneous humor, on the other hand, arises out of ordinary situations and is usually a witty remark inspired by the circumstances at hand. Its success depends on the right moment and right circle of participants.[1]

Spontaneous humor is further defined as "jocular remarks" which consist of two forms: pleasantries and witticisms.

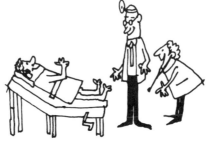

A pleasantry is a mild form of humor to which no laughter may be attached. It may be simply a humorous turn of phrase, an attempt to be pleasant by being mildly amusing rather than definitely trying to entertain. A witticism, on the other hand, makes a greater attempt to entertain. It is more clever and original. "Pleasantries are little bubbles coming to the surface of the water and disappearing, a witticism makes a loud splash."[2]

William Fry has provided a similar division. He defines spontaneous humor as situation jokes, which have their origin in the ongoing interpersonal process. Canned jokes are those presented with little obvious relationship to the ongoing human interaction. Practical jokes are a combination of both, in that they are consciously contrived but depend on the unfolding of an interpersonal interaction for the humor to occur.[3]

The use of both spontaneous and formal humor will be discussed in the sections on *Humor in Health and Illness* and *Cultivating the Use of Humor.*

REFERENCES

1. Emerson, *Humor in Hospital Settings,* pp 11-12.
2. *Ibid,* p 137.
3. Fry, *Sweet Madness,* pp 41-43.

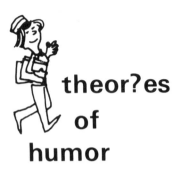

theor?es
of
humor

Despite the lack of consensus as to theory and despite the formidable task of attempting to review all the literature, I am as undaunted, and as apologetic, as all the previous authors! In the absence of a single framework to which to relate, not having this overall background knowledge would seem to be like embarking on a trip without a map.

However, this chapter only attempts an overview to provide a perspective for the development of the major thesis of this book, since many of the theories and studies will be discussed in detail in other chapters in relation to specific areas. For those who wish even greater depth, the original works are, of course, available. (If however, you are a free spirit who prefers to travel unburdened by maps, you are at liberty to move on!)

Many of the writings about humor have not offered pure theories as such. Many of them have included analyses of specific characteristics of humor. Many have been speculations as to the nature of humor or the functions of humor. Many are classics in the field but have cogent points to make which add to the understanding of humor and so are included in any discussion of theory. However, this multifaceted approach poses problems in a categorization of theories. Consequently, three approaches have been used. One has been to do a chronological, historical accounting by years or centuries. A second method is to categorize by discipline: philosophy, comedy writing and critique, psychology, psychoanalysis, anthropology and sociology. The third approach is by functional or issue categories. I shall summarize from each of the last two approaches.

PHILOSOPHICAL PERSPECTIVES

Early philosophers were primarily concerned with the nature of humor in relation to the nature of man, and the issue of good and evil. Does humor represent the best in man or the worst? Plato and Aristotle felt that humor was enjoyment of the misfortune of others and comedy was an imitation of men at their worst. Others have viewed laughter as a weapon against evil and a valuable asset in correcting minor follies of society.

PERSPECTIVES OF COMEDY WRITERS AND CRITICS

Comedy writers and critics have also been concerned with the nature of comedy. Comedy reveals man's imperfections, leaves him more tolerant, and gives him the courage to face life; this is the theme of most comedy writers and comedians. Comedy is not just a happy as opposed to an unhappy ending, but a way of surveying life. All tragedy is idealistic and says "the pity of it," while comedy tends to be skeptical and says, "the absurdity of it."

> In mortal affairs it is tragedy, like forgiveness, that seems divine, and comedy, like error, that is human.[1]

Elements of comedy and styles of humor, *i.e.,* what makes people laugh and how can one create it, has been the major focus of others.

PSYCHOANALYTIC PERSPECTIVES

The psychoanalytic theory of humor originated by Sigmund Freud has been perhaps one of the major frameworks for the study of humor in recent years. Freud became interested in jokes when he became aware of the similarity between the technique of jokes and dreams, resulting in his book, *Jokes and their Relation to the Unconscious* (1905).[2] There are two types of jokes: the harmless joke, and the joke with a purpose or "tendentious" wit. Civilization has produced repression of many basic impulses, he says, and joking is a socially acceptable way of satisfying these needs. He describes four types of purposeful jokes: the sexual joke; the aggressive, hostile joke; the blasphemous joke; and the skeptical joke. The process is an unconscious one and there is a saving of psychic energy.

Freud differentiates between wit, the comic effect, and humor. However, all have the same motif, that of economy. The pleasure of wit originates from the economy of inhibition, the comic from the economy of thought, and humor from an economy of feelings. This effect strives to reproduce the state of childhood when our expenditure of psychic energy was slight and we did not need all these jokes, humor, and comic effects to "make us feel happy in our life."

Freud also developed a theory of laughing at tragedy and death, called "gallows humor," which has been the basis for much study since and will be discussed later in relation to medical humor.

In a short article published in 1928, Freud further

developed his concept of humor.[3] Humor has something liberating about it, is not resigned. The ego refuses to be distressed by reality, to let itself suffer. It is a triumph of narcissism through the indulgence of the superego, yet does not overstep the bounds of mental health. Not everyone, he says, is capable of this rare and precious gift, however.

Many of the studies and other thinking since then have been built on Freud's base.

PSYCHOLOGICAL PERSPECTIVES

The psychologists have concerned themselves more with the individual in relation to humor, *i.e.*, why one individual laughs and not another. They have also focused on laboratory-controlled experiments rather than arm-chair theorizing or studies in natural settings. They have looked at such personality traits as aggression, sex, creativity, and intelligence, among others, in relation to humor as well as to the presence or development of a "sense of humor." Much of this work has used Freud's theory as a base.

More recently, psychologists have become concerned with the lack of any systematic empirical and theoretical attack on humor and have voiced the belief that, although psychoanalytic theory has made a significant contribution, it is limited in its capacity to stimulate further advancement.[4] The new approach is built around arousal and cognitive factors. Humor is not simply determined by the present stimulus situation but depends on recollections of the past and anticipations of the future. It is a collative process which is important in generating or arousing the pleasure of humor. The processing of these collative properties is cognitively based; it also involves information-processing and problem-solving ability. We must perceive the incongruity and resolve it before we "get the joke."

Harvey Mindess proposes another theory he calls liberation theory in which he sees humor as the agent of psychological liberation. It frees us from the constraints and restrictive forces of daily living and in so doing makes us joyful. His theory, he says, encompasses all the others. He urges us to cultivate our sense of humor and provides us with some thoughts on how to achieve this.

ANTHROPOLOGICAL PERSPECTIVES

The main contributions of the anthropologists have been to describe the humor components within cultures or ethnic groups as a part of their investigations. Radcliffe-Brown's early (1940) identification of the joking relationships between kin members greatly influenced other research. He defined the joking relationship as a:

> ....relation between two persons in which one is by custom permitted, and, in some instances required, to tease or make fun of the other, who in turn is required to take no offense.[6]

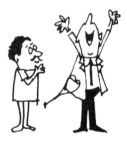

It is one of "permitted disrespect," a combination of friendliness and antagonism. This kind of social relationship is widespread in other societies and the concept provides a base for comparative studies of social structures.

Extensive studies of humor in the Navajo culture are perhaps the most well known, and describe the Navajo as having a keen sense of humor. Studies of humor in other cultures have not been extensively researched. Crosscultural studies of humor are also needed.

SOCIOLOGICAL PERSPECTIVES

Although the sociologists have been the last group to get involved in the concept of humor, their contributions have been increasing. Perhaps the first sociological theory was offered in 1900 by Henri Bergson who described the nature of humor as "the mechanical encrusted on the living." A person is laughable when he behaves in a rigid, automatic, routinized way. Humor functions as a social corrective on this unadaptive behavior. The comic, Bergson says, does not exist outside the pale of the human. Laughter is always within a group and must remain in touch with other intelligences. Laughter functions to socialize the individual into a group and groups into society.

Others credit Obrdlik's article on the phenomenon of gallows humor in Nazi-occupied Czechoslovakia as the first to deal with humor in a sociological framework.[8] The humor served a social function in bolstering morale of the oppressed group while disintegrating the forces against whom the humor was directed. The humor made the fear and tragedy seem temporary.

Studies of the social functions of humor in race relations and in ethnic and minority groups (the Negro was studied by many) describe the function of humor to solidify the in-group, to attain gratification at the expense of another group, and, more recently, as a way to create a new image and as an agent for social change. The role of the fool in society has been described as a lowly one, yet valued. The fool serves as a scapegoat, and as a means of enforcing group norms of propriety. Others have also emphasized the control function of humor as a means of expressing approval or disapproval of social actions and to relieve tension in social conflict. The social functions and joking relationships in organizations which serve to minimize the strain and release antagonism and the social functions of humor within the hospital setting have also been studied.

BIOLOGICAL AND INSTINCT THEORIES

Many theorists have viewed laughter as a physiologic mechanism which is "good for the body." McDougall believed that laughter was basically an instinct invented by nature as an antidote to our tendency to sympathize with the distresses of others.[9] Laughter produces a physiologic sense of well-being and a euphoria which has a biologic "survival" value. Secondarily, he says, laughter serves a social function in that the sense of humor makes us capable of laughing at our own minor misfortunes. There is also a larger humor, which finds laughter in those defects common to all men. Koestler also describes laughter as a physiological reaction similar to tears, which seem to have no biological function yet produce such obvious relief that they can hardly be called "luxury reflexes."[10] Koestler goes on to link laughter with comedy and describes comedy as an act of creativity. Others have described laughter as an evolutionary process beginning with the "baring of teeth" and snarling to forestall attack and developing into the smile and laugh which communicates that one can relax in safety. Laughter and humor have become a substitute for actual assault.

SUPERIORITY THEORIES

The basis of the superiority theory lies in the assertion of our own superiority by laughing at the inferiority, stupidity, or misfortunes of others. Plato and Aristotle reflected this pleasure in the pain of others. Hobbes defined laughter as a "sudden glory arising from some sudden conception of some eminency in ourselves by comparison with the infirmity of others." Bergson's theory of "the mechanical encrusted on the living" views humor as laughing at the stereotyped, unsocial behavior of others. Ridicule and laughter at the foolish actions of others are reflected in the clown, Charlie Chaplin, Laurel and Hardy, the Keystone Kops, the pie-in-the-face, slipping-on-a-banana-peel type of comedy. Others believe that this laughter is not always cruel or scornful, but that it may be a laughter of warmth, sympathy, and empathy as well. It may also reflect a laughing at our own inferiorities.

SURPRISE, INCONGRUITY, AMBIVALENCE, OR CONFLICT THEORIES

These words have been used interchangeably by various authors to describe a necessary element or component of the humorous experience. There must be a "surprise," a sudden "shock" or unexpectedness, an incongruity, ambivalence, or conflict of ideas or emotions which produces the absurdity or ludicrousness resulting in a burst of laughter.

Kant observed that laughter is "an affection arising from the sudden transformation of a strained expectation into nothing." For Schopenhauer, laughter arises from the sudden perception of an incongruity between an object and a concept. Spencer saw laughter occurring when "the conscious is unawares transferred from great things to small — a descending incongruity." An ascending incongruity gives rise to wonder, not laughter. Bergson stated that a situation is comic when it belongs simultaneously to two altogether independent series of events and is capable of being interpreted in two entirely different meanings at the same time. Koestler attributed humor to "biosociation," perceiving a situation or event in two habitually incompatible associated contexts.

Monro described the experience of ambivalent emotions. We laugh whenever, on contemplating an object or situation, we find opposite emotions struggling within us for mastery.[11]

Many other authors in their writings have also identified this concept of surprise or incongruity as the necessary ingredient in the creation of humor.

CONFIGURATIONAL THEORIES

These theories are similar to the surprise and incongruity theories except that it is the sudden "insight" or "falling into place" that creates the laughter rather than the unexpected "disjointedness" that is the amusement of incongruity.

Configurational theories are based on the broader theoretical model of Gestalt psychology which involves perception of the whole. We begin ordering perceptions in a reasoning fashion when they are presented, but it is the unexpected configuration which results that is the surprise and appears ludicrous. The appreciation of a joke has been related to shifts in figure-ground perception. When the reversal occurs, we "get the point" of the joke.

RELIEF OR RELEASE THEORIES

Many theories have as their base the concept of humor as a relief from tension, anxiety, and frustration or the release from the harsh realities of life. Freud's theory essentially falls into this category as well as the liberation theory of Mindess. Many other theorists have incorporated the idea of relief as one of the functions of humor into their theories.

PLAY THEORIES

Many writers have described humor as an aspect of play, made comparisons between play and humor, or incorporated the aspect of play as a developmental factor in acquiring a sense of humor. The "playful" nature of humor and laughter is common to most theories of the nature of humor.

Sully stated that the enjoyment of the laughable comes from arousal of the play mood, a refusal to take the situation seriously, which is the characteristic feature of play.[12] Laughter prepares us for social life in a manner similar to play.

Eastman defined humor as play, stating humor has no value except the values possessed by play. No definition or explanation of humor will hold up, he says, which is not based on a distinction between playful and serious. He discusses the strange phenomenon of tickling as associated with play and laughter.

William Fry has done an extensive study of the relation of humor to play, and laughing and smiling to both.[14] Both involve an interpersonal interaction communication, both are sensitive to the spontaneity-thoughtfulness balance, and both involve manipulation in the levels of abstraction. Fry describes the development of play and humor from birth to adulthood. He describes both as having to have a framework of unreality or fun, i.e., a play-frame and a joke frame. He also compares play and humor to fighting and aggression — the wrestling around and playful slaps are related to the "punch" line of the joke.

Berlyne, in his discussion of laughter, humor, and play, states that laughter and play are so widespread in human societies that their absence may be judged abnormal.[15] As a matter of fact, societies expend a greater part of their time and energy in playful and humorous pursuits.

SUMMARY

It should be apparent after this brief review why this concept of humor is still so controversial. For so common a phenomenon, it is extremely complex! Most of the theories have yet to be empirically tested. Yet the paradox of seriously studying humor has already been described. In looking at theories, the only solution seems to be to remain as open and eclectic as possible in trying to understand this vital human behavior!

REFERENCES

1. Kronenberger L: Some prefatory words on comedy. *In* Felheim M (ed): *Comedy,* p 194.
2. Freud S: Jokes and their relation to the unconscious (1905), vol VIII. *In* Strachey J. (ed): *The Complete Psychological Works of Sigmund Freud.* London, Hogarth Press, 1961.
3. Freud, S: *Humour,* vol XXI. 1927 pp 160-166.
4. Goldstein JH; McGhee PE: *The Psychology of Humor.* New York, NY, Academic Press, 1972.
5. Mindess, *Laughter and Liberation,* 1971.
6. Radcliffe-Brown AR: *Structure and Function in Primitive Society.* New York, NY, The Free Press, 1965 p 90.
7. Bergson H: Laughter: *In* Enck JJ: Forter ET, Whitley A. (eds): pp 43-64.
8. Obrdlik, AJ: Gallows humor, a sociological phenomenon. *American Journal of Sociology* 47:709-716, 1942.
9. McDougall W: An instinct of laughter. (1903) *An Introduction to Social Psychology.* New York, NY, University Paperbacks, Barnes and Noble, 1963.
10. Koestler A: *The Act of Creation.* New York, The Macmillan Co, 1964.
11. Monro DH: *Argument of Laughter.* Melbourne, Melbourne University Press, 1951.
12. Sully J.: Essay on laughter (1902). *In* Piddington R: *The Psychology of Laughter: A Study in Social Adaptation.* New York, Gamut Press, 1963, pp 196-200.
13. Eastman M: *The Enjoyment of Laughter.* New York, Simon and Schuster, 1936.
14. Fry, *Sweet Madness,* 1963.
15. Berlyne DE: Laughter, humor and play. *Handbook of Social Psychology* 3:795-813, 1969.

BIBLIOGRAPHY

Flugel JC: Humor and laughter. *In* Lindsay G (ed): *Handbook of Social Psychology II.* Cambridge, Mass Addison-Wesley, 1954, pp 709-734.
Keith-Spiegel P: Early conceptions of humor: varieties and issues. *In* Goldstein JH; McGhee PE (eds): *The Psychology of Humor,* 1971, pp 3-39.

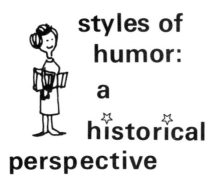

styles of humor: a ⭐historical⭐ perspective

Another of the complexities in studying the concepts of humor is in the style of the comedy itself. A review of the literature of comedy reveals one very striking note: the style of the humor varies tremendously. From Aristophanes to Chaucer, to Moliere, to Shakespeare, to Mark Twain, to Will Rogers, to Joseph Heller and Bob Hope, the range of comedy is almost overwhelming. It is obvious that the social and political climate, the historical events and situation of any particular era or time in history affect the style of the humor. What is viewed as hilarious by one generation may be completely unfunny and not understandable to another.

There are some classic comedies which have survived over the years, but these very often must be interpreted to be appreciated.

> Though comedy has its permanent subject matter and even its body of laws, it is liable, like everything else to changes in fashion and taste, to differences of sensibility. One generation's pleasure is the next generation's embarrassment. Much that the Victorians shuddered at merely makes us laugh...[1]

It is interesting to note, however, that George Meredith in his famous lecture on comedy in 1877, reflecting the thought of the Victorian age, stated that comedy requires a society of cultivated men and women in a civilization that has some degree of social equality of the sexes!

> ...where they have no social freedom, comedy is absent; where they are household drudges, the form of comedy is primitive....But where women are on the road to an equal footing with men...there...pure comedy flourishes.[2]

Bonamy Dobree contends that:

> ...in the history of dramatic literature there are some periods labelled as definitely "tragic," others as no less preponderatingly "comic," though of course, both forms exist side by side throughout the ages.[3]

Tragedy thrives in periods of great national expansion and power, during which values are fixed and positive. In great "comic" periods, values are changing; the times are ones of rapid social readjustment and general instability, when policy is insecure, religion doubted and being revised, and morality in a state of chaos. However, the greatest names in comedy, Aristophanes, Jonson, and Moliere, flourished in the intermediate periods when tragedy has lost its positive character and men begin to doubt if the old values are, after all, the best.

American humor has had its periods of style and change. The frontier spirit, the need for cunning and strength for survival, and a simple homely philosophy were reflected in our American humor. It started with the exaggerations of the first settlers who came over against the advice of family and friends and were anxious to make good. Exaggeration is the foundation of the tall tales and stories of Paul Bunyan, Davy Crockett, and, later, Mark Twain.

When the Western migration spilled over the Alleghenies and beyond, the peculiar brand of humor called Midwestern sprang up. The Midwestern frontier was a new experience and often a rude shock. Laughter was the only relief. The humor was often "uncouth, boastful, bombastic, and irreverent." It loved to puncture illusions, pretensions of grandeur and snobbishness. The "sucker" or victim of practical jokes became the comic figure from the "tenderfoot" to the "simple soul." Out of the Midwest came a fantastic array of literary humorists; Mark Twain, Booth Tarkington, Damon Runyon, Ring Lardner, and James Thurber are examples. Other Midwest comedians include Will Rogers, Red Skelton, Clifton Webb, Joe E. Brown, Buster Keaton, Harold Lloyd, Jack Benny, Bob Hope, and Herb Shriner.

The Roaring Twenties and early Thirties were considered by many to be the Golden Age of Humor. That period spawned such comedians as Charlie Chaplin, Laurel and Hardy, the Marx Brothers, Robert Benchley, Will Rogers, and W.C. Fields.

However, from the Thirties through the Sixties there was a stalemate in this kind of honest healthy humor. People were too stunned by the harsh realities to laugh at absurdities. This was the time of depression, war, assassinations, racial riots, and campus revolutions. When you are shooting down the system it is difficult to laugh at it. The jokes of the period reflected this tension. There were first the empty jokes — the Shaggy Dog stories, the "Knock-Knock, Who's There?", and the Elephant jokes. There were also the scapegoat jokes — the Polack jokes, the monster jokes, and the sick jokes. Bergan Evans, speaking of the Sixties, called it the age of the bland and characterized the comedians as the "bland leading the bland." He felt people were so insecure they could not bear to be laughed at or to laugh at themselves. It was not a time for satire. Satire, which Evans defines as the "art of being nasty" or the "Sword of Wit," is a type of humor which is not intended for the masses. Satire is civilized, controlled rage, alien to the popular mind which expresses its emotions more directly. Pope and Swift wrote for less than 1 percent of the population, the "literate."

There arose, however, a technique of comedy writing

coined by Bruce Jay Friedman as "black humor," a grotesque absurdist humor similar in many respects to the "gallows" humor described by Freud and the "medical" humor of the health professionals. This particular style will be examined further in a later chapter.

Comedians of today, the Seventies, feel that we are in a new age of humor, one that is honest and reflective, and in which we are beginning to be able to laugh at ourselves again. It is a healthy sign. To be able to laugh at oneself and the foibles of mankind is a sign of maturity. It is a "renaissance of laughter."

> ...we have come through the dark '60s craving humor.... When you've got that many people angry you've either got to hit, leave, or laugh. We can't leave, and we've tried hitting. Laughter is all that's left (*The Denver Post,* April 10, 1972).

The new humor was borne in on the waves of television's *Laugh-In.* Satire has had a revival through Art Buchwald, Archie Bunker, and stand-up comedians like Mort Sahl. What the satirist is blessed with today, Buchwald says, is an informed and intelligent audience. Reality is the basis for comedy and, like new strengths which result from coping with crisis, out of times of tension and turmoil and changing values arises some of the best humor.

Humor about health and illness and health professionals has followed the styles of the era or times also. A book entitled *Wit and Humor of the Age* written in 1883 by Melville D. Landon, has a chapter entitled "Doctors, Wit and Humor." The following reflects the "homespun" quality of that era.

> My doctor, Dr. Hammond, is a great doctor. He can cure cholory or smallpox, or hams or bacon.
>
> One day I cut off my toe with an axe. When I called in Dr. Hammond to prescribe for me he told me to hold out my tongue. He said he thought I had tic doloro, and then he prescribed bleeding, and then he bled me out of seventeen dollars. That was the dollar, and when he wanted his pay I told him to charge it, and that was the tic, and I still owe it to him, and that is the "o."[4]

Although medical treatment has changed, complaints about medical fees apparently have not!

The humor of the Forties brought with it the lampooning of the medical and nursing profession with stories and cartoons in the professional journals themselves. "The Probie," the probationer student nurse, was the butt of much humor, and revealed the anxieties of the professional.

"Quick, pick it up off the floor before it gets unsterile."

A student with a tray full of dentures collected from patients, says to the head nurse, "Now what do I do?"

Richard Armour satirizes the medical profession:

> *The Doctor's Life*
> Look up noses,
>   Look down throats,
> Look up nostrums,
>   Jot down notes,
>
> Look up rectums,
>   Look down ears,
> Look up patients
>   In arrears,
>
> Pull down covers,
>   Pull up gowns....
> Life is full of
>   Ups and downs.[5]

Today's humorous get-well cards, jokes about psychiatrists, novels, and TV shows demonstrate that not only is the public more knowledgeable about health and disease, but also more comfortable in poking fun at it.

A Little Learning

Patients once let surgeons cut
Without an if or and or but.
They rarely raised demanding questions
And never offered up suggestions.

Patients once, not long ago,
Believed the doctor ought to know,
Submitted with the best of will,
And trusted in his practiced skill.

But patients now, and patients' wives,
Are sharper than a surgeon's knives,
And argue over each incision....
They've seen it all on television.[6]

REFERENCES

1. Kronenberger L: Some prefatory words. *In* Felheim, p 197.
2. Meredith G: On comedy and the uses of the comic spirit. *In* Felheim (ed): p 210.
3. Dobree B: Restoration comedy, drama and values. *In* Felheim (ed), p 202.
4. Landon MD: *Wit and Humor of the Age.* Chicago, Star Publishing Co, 1883, p 436.
5. Armour R: *The Medical Muse.* New York: McGraw-Hill Book Co, 1963, p 3.
6. *Ibid,* p 33.

BIBLIOGRAPHY

Brown J: *Perennially Yours, Probie.* New York Springer Publishing Co, 1958.
Harrel S: *When It's Laughter You're After.* Norman, Oklahoma, University of Oklahoma Press, 1962, chapter 9.

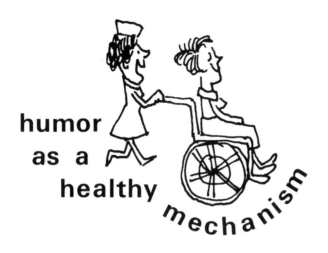

humor as a healthy mechanism

The basic assumption or framework upon which this study is built is the belief that humor is a form of human behavior that is healthy and constructive. Yet, despite the recognition that humorous pursuits are a widespread activity in almost all human societies — and the preponderance of authors and investigators who attest to its value — the question as to whether humor is healthy or unhealthy continues to arise and that issue is a source of debate (along with all the other issues!).

Questions are always asked in relation to the "uncontrollable" laughter of hysteria, the "inappropriate" laughter of the mentally ill, and the motivation behind hostile satirical humor, the black humor and sick jokes.

Keith-Spiegel, discussing this controversy, points out three possibilities in the healthy-unhealthy dimension.[1] Is the laughing, joking person (1) revealing that he is healthy and mentally well-balanced, or (2) divulging his innermost hang-ups and deep-seated problems, or (3) since he is laughing, indicating that he is handling his mental conflicts and worries in a healthy manner by converting them to pleasure? Some authors have focused on just one aspect, but most theorists have spanned all three dimensions in their writings.

Freud's concept of joking was based on his original theory of repression and unconscious conflicts. That which we laugh at is indicative of our problems or inhibitions. But, Freud contends, joking becomes a healthy and socially adaptive way of handling these problems. He goes on to compare humor to other more pathological methods used by the human mind, namely, neuroses, psychoses, intoxication, etc. Yet, humor he says, manages the same effect "without overstepping the bounds of mental health."[2] He further states that not everyone is capable of this humorous attitude, that it is a rare and precious gift.

Martin Grotjahn, in his interpretation of humor and laughter based on Freud's theory, contends that Freud did not go deep enough into the aggressive, hostile aspects of humor. Grotjahn speaks of wit as related to aggression, hostility, and sadism, and humor as related to depression, narcissism, and masochism. He describes the wit, the tease, the kidder, the practical joker, the cynic, the clown as belonging to that large family of people struggling to find a permissible outlet for their aggressions and/or also avoiding depression. A devastating analysis! Yet, he contrasts these characterizations with the statements that "a sense of humor signifies emotional maturity," and "laughter is a sign of strength, freedom, health, beauty, youth, and happiness." There is a need, he says, for this free and episodic regression in order to gain strength for this reality we live in.[3]

McDougall describes laughter as a biological instinct devised by nature as an antidote for the depression and pain we feel in sympathizing with the overwhelming misfortunes or miseries of others. It has "survival value." He goes on to describe a —

> ...larger humor which finds occasion for laughter in those defects and shortcomings which are common to all men; such humor including in its object the laugher himself, does not wound, as does the lower, simpler form of laughter; for it brings a bond of fellowship between him who laughs and all his fellows, inviting all men, without discrimination, to share in the genial exercise. Humorous laughter is thus a higher form which implies the attainment in some degree of the power of viewing ourselves objectively, of seeing ourselves as others see us.[4]

Are these seemingly disparate thoughts contradictions? Or do they merely reinforce again the paradoxical nature of humor and laughter? Essentially, humor ranges on a continuum, and it becomes obvious that each individual's "sense of humor" is related to his own needs, personality, and point in time. There is no absolute positive or negative aspect to humor.

This very issue of healthy and unhealthy humor is comparable to the problem of defining health and mental health which has occupied the time and concern of health professionals for many years. What is health and what is mental health? How does one know when they have been achieved? Conversely, what is disease or mental illness? The conclusions reached are that health is not merely the absence of disease, but, that health and illness range on a continuum, and each is a dynamic process of adaptation and adjustment to maintain homeostasis or a balance. Perfect health and perfect mental health are illusions. We have established criteria and characteristics for both, but in reality no one ever achieves that ultimate. Rather, we recognize that health is an individual state and "wellness" is defined in terms of each person's maximizing his potential and functioning to his own optimal level.

This recognition has influenced the therapeutic

measures and the professional's role toward a more humanistic approach to the achievement of health.

We have also recognized that stress, stemming either internally from within the individual or externally from the environment in which he lives, creates physiological changes within the human organism, and, therefore, physical health and mental health are inextricably intertwined.

Humor and laughter, as a form of human behavior which is defined on the one hand as a biological, physiological reflex and on the other hand as a psychological, adaptive, defense mechanism, share this same phenomenon. The physiological changes produced by laughter have been described as stimulating respiration and circulation and decreasing hypertension, leading to a feeling of well-being. The relief from anxiety and tension which laughter and humor can accomplish reverses the harmful physiological changes caused by the anxiety. Studies have shown that reduction of anxiety prior to surgery has facilitated postoperative recovery and has reduced postoperative complications. Is not the use of humor as a way of coping with aggression and anger "health-producing" for the individual?

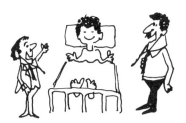

Particularly, if it reduces hypertension and prevents depression! Theodore Reik once quipped, "A murderous thought a day keeps the doctor away!" Certainly, it must be "health-producing" for the individual toward whom the murderous rage is directed! Konrad Lorenz, in discussing the value of humor, says, "Barking dogs may occasionally bite, but laughing men hardly ever shoot!"[5]

George Mikes points out that humor keeps man in a sense of proportion, that even though laughter and humor can be aggressive and have a malicious intent, there is reason for cherishing these offensive elements.[6] Human nature, he says, is not peerless and angelic and one needs to get rid of a certain amount of nastiness, so why not laugh it off? Even the most aggressive jokes are better than the least aggressive wars.

In summary, humor ranges on a continuum from healthy to unhealthy. It is healthy when it deals with immediate issues and helps the individual handle realities. It becomes destructive and dysfunctional only when it abets pathological denial of reality — when it becomes a running-away from the difficulties of living rather than an easing of the way to deal with the "heavies" of living.

This aspect of reality-unreality is inherent in the issue of healthy versus unhealthy. The very "play" nature of humor implies a fantasy, an absurd, ludicrous situation which is "not real." "This is a joke." Yet, the reality or seriousness of the content of the joke must be evident and intelligible for the listener to "get the point."

Humor is very honest, yet avoids serious implications by placing the comment in a joke frame. William Fry discusses extensively the real-unreal paradox and describes the purpose of the "punch line" as projecting the implicit materials within the joke into the "workaday world" of reality.[7] Humor, says Lorenz, is the "best of lie-detectors." "It discovers with an uncanny flair, the speciousness of contrived ideals and the insincerity of simulated enthusiasm."[8] Thus, humor tends to make the world a more honest place.

Other authors have pointed out that one of the important functions of humor is to relieve us of the burdens of reality. The enjoyment of humor rests upon a make-believe world wherein all the rules of logic, time, place, reality, and proper conduct are suspended. Even sheer nonsense and absurdity are a way to take one's thoughts away from the seriousness of living and provide a feeling that life is not so overwhelmingly tragic. The extent of this reality-unreality within each humorous situation, of course, will vary, but this element exists as another component in the complexity of the concept.

Another closely related element is the repression-liberation issue. Do we laugh most loudly at those things about which we are the most inhibited and have problems, or do we laugh more easily at those things about which we feel more liberated and comfortable? There are viewpoints at either end of this continuum. Does the "inhibited" staid "old maid" really laugh louder at sexual jokes than does the "sexually free" individual? The psychoanalytic theorists have built their case on the repression model. Others claim, like Mindess, that, our sense of humor simply "frees us from all the constraints of conventionality, morality, reason and other restrictive forces."[9] However, can one be liberated without having been inhibited or restricted in some way? There is probably a continuum here also, depending again on the content, individual, and situation.

Other continuums evidence themselves within this framework of healthy-unhealthy.

There is obviously a range from an immature, more childlike "laughing at" to a more mature "laughing with." Many authors make a great distinction between these. Wit, practical jokes, slapstick comedy, the tease, the clown, the superiority-inferiority jokes fall at the "laughing at" end of the continuum. McDougall's "larger humor," Freud's liberating humor and the humor of the self-actualized man which Abraham Maslow describes as a "humor of the real," a thoughtful philosophic humor, falls at the "laughing with" end of the continuum.

The functions or purposes or needs which humor serves also range on a continuum from simple nonsense pleasure to warmth, to social needs, to anxieties, to

34

anger, and to the deeper psychological needs around tragedy and death. The kinds of humor and the styles of humor also vary to meet these needs, ranging from nonsense jokes, pleasantries, and witticisms to satire and gallows humor.

Within the life and death arena of the health and illness settings these continuums are very evident. Because of the unique nature of this setting, unlike society in general, there are far more instances at the tragedy end of the continuum. It becomes necessary then to look very closely at the use of humor in this context. Whose needs are being met and how? The emotionality of these tragedies affect the professional as well as the patient and his family. If the professional is to use humor as a therapeutic tool, he must be aware of all the issues and the continuums in the nature of humor.

This framework of the nature of humor will be the basis upon which we will explore the uses of humor within health-illness settings in *Section II* and the assumptions set forth in *Section III* in cultivating the use of humor as a therapeutic tool.

REFERENCES

1. Keith-Spiegel, P: Early conceptions of humor: varieties and issues. *In* Goldstein JH, McGhee PE (ed): *The Psychology of Humor,* p 28.
2. Freud S: *Humor,* p 163.
3. Grotjahn, *Beyond Laughter,* pp. 255-264.
4. McDougall, *An Instinct of Laughter,* p 395.
5. Lorenz K: *On Aggression.* New York, Harcourt, Brace and World, 1963, p 285.
6. Mikes G: *Laughing Matter.* New York, The Library Press, 1971.
7. Fry, *Sweet Madness,* p 152.
8. Lorenz, *On Aggression,* p 287.
9. Mindess, *Laughter and Liberation,* p 241.

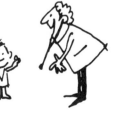

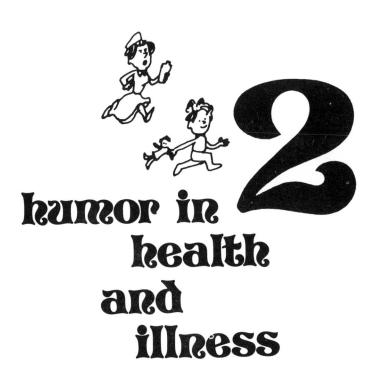

humor in health and illness

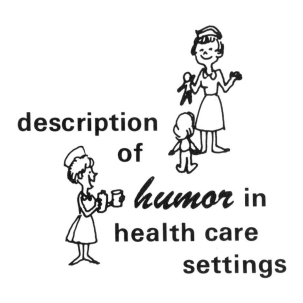

description of *humor* in health care settings

Humor is a familiar pattern of communication which both health professionals and patients bring with them into the health care setting. However, humor is not considered to be a formal communication mode. Rather, it is an indirect form of communication, one which is casual and inconspicuously blended into the general flow of events. Because health and illness are "serious" business, humor is not an expected occurrence. Despite this, humor is permitted and actually occurs in almost any situation.

This "optional" and not expected quality may be a contributing factor to the meagerness of studies and descriptions of humor in this setting as well as other natural settings. Of the three major sociological studies which have reported observations of humor in hospitals, none was originally designed to study humor specifically as it relates to health.

Two studies were serendipitous. Rose Laub Coser set out to study the social structure of a hospital ward and the role of the patient in it. Her observations of humor and jocular talk led to the formulation of some valuable hypotheses.[1] Renee Fox's study was designed to investigate an experimental metabolic ward and the social process of physicians and patients facing uncertainties and unknowns.[2] She discovered that a highly patterned and intricate form of joking and humor was one of the most important ways both physicians and patients evolved for coming to terms with the stresses of facing death.

On the other hand, the third study, conducted by Joan Emerson, was a doctoral dissertation conceived as a step in the systematic investigation of the sociology of humor, but was not concerned with hospitals as such.[3] She chose a general hospital as her natural setting because it was a large organization with a distinct status hierarchy and structured interaction. One of her goals was to show how the nature of humor is related to the structural problems of the setting in which it occurs. She chose two particular "delicate" situations upon which to focus: the pelvic examination and death.

All three provided invaluable insights and contributions to the understanding of humor in health settings and are the basis for this author's study.[4] However, they point out the need for more definitive and rigorous investigation. Humor in health settings has been serendipitous long enough!

Within this unique world of health and illness, humor serves three major functions: a communication function, a social function, and a psychological function. Humor serves to communicate important messages, to promote social relations, and to diminish the discomforts and manage the "delicate" situations which occur in this setting. A big order for such an indirect and casual phenomenon! The three functions, of course, are intertwined in any situation. Humor originates internally but requires an audience and must be communicated!

Communication

The messages which need to be communicated within the hospital or other health setting are usually very serious and emotion-laden: anxiety, fear, embarrassment, anger, tragedy, concern, hope, and joy. Yet their direct expression is not always acceptable or comfortable. Humor serves to convey these in an indirect fashion, and, because of its play frame, provides a vehicle for moving easily in or out of the "serious" as the situation warrants.

In time of illness, strangers (patients and staff) are thrown together, very suddenly, into very intimate and somber contacts. There is no time to build up a relationship. Individuals must interact without much knowledge about each other and with no expectancy of a continuing relationship once the immediate health crisis is resolved. The patient must trust the health professional and accept his competency and concern almost on faith. The professional also expects the patient, almost without question, to cooperate with and submit to very intimate, foreboding procedures and treatments.

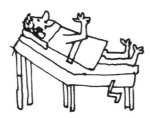

A form of interaction which very quickly provides a sense of familiarity, does not offend, and is easily facilitated is needed. Humor meets these criteria and is highly suitable for this kind of interaction. Joan Emerson found that pleasantries around standard topics established this sense of familiarity among the participants in the hospital interactions she observed.[5] This mild form of humor, including banter and jocular talk, provides the flexibility for easily terminating the interaction or moving into more "serious" humor and/or a serious discussion.

In a typical hospital ward, where a number of persons are approaching the patient for a variety of reasons and where "any encounter is highly subject to interruption," there is a need to be able to disrupt an interaction without creating ill feelings. The reverse is also possible. This indirect form of communication provides a convenient stepping stone for transmitting more serious concerns. The more highly charged humor with "serious import" could also lead to overt discussion of those matters, if the transition is acceptable. If there is not time to negotiate this or the patient is not ready, however, it is very easy to retreat since humor is "not really serious business." The laughter or smile of the recipient acknowledges that he has received the implicit message in the joking. Often, just knowing that others know you are frightened or anxious or angry is a release in itself, and the fact that the message was conveyed often suffices.

As William Fry stated so succinctly, a joke has a host of unconscious chords which sound in the audience's mind no less loudly than does the explicit joke. This, he says, proves the vital link between humor and life. "By these bridges of the unconscious the stream between humor and life is crossed and recrossed, and there is found to be ample traffic from shore to shore."[6]

SOCIAL FUNCTIONS

Humor serves a valuable purpose in "promoting the continued harmony of a social relation at the same time that important messages are conveyed."[7]

The hospital society is one in which many of the rules of the normal society are disrupted, violated, or suspended. The patient is placed in a dependent role, his privacy is invaded, and the normal social relationships and behavior to which he is accustomed are often waived. Humor provides a mechanism for coping with these disruptive social acts. It assists in establishing relationships, releases tension from the social conflicts, promotes solidarity, provides social control, and manages those "delicate" situations created by illness and the hospital structure.

Establishing Relationships

Humor is used frequently to establish the necessary relationships within the health setting. It breaks the ice, reduces fear of the unfamiliar setting, encourages a sense of trust, and establishes a feeling of camaraderie and of friendship. It says to the patient, or colleague or student, "Relax. I'm a friend, you can trust me. This isn't such a terrible place." It sets the tone for a more relaxed atmosphere, much as the main speaker at a dinner does with his introductory joke or humorous comment.

> When a male patient who was admitted for a biopsy was sent to a gynecological ward because of a shortage of beds, the nurses teased him with, "You're in for a hysterectomy, of course!" and "You're the only male on the ward and I thought we were liberated!"

The patient, on admission to this strange and unknown environment will joke about "all the hotel service" he'll be getting and the "pretty nurses to take care of him." Rose Laub Coser stated: "to laugh, or to occasion laughter through humor and wit, is to invite those present to come closer...it aims at decreasing social distance."[8] She goes on to say that the contribution humor makes to social economy within the institution of the hospital should be stressed.

> In such a shifting and threatening milieu, a story well told, which, in a few minutes, entertains, reassures, conveys information, releases tension, and draws people more closely together, may have more to contribute than carefully planned lectures and discussions toward the security of the frightened sick.[9]

In this highly structured organization where there is a definite status hierarchy with the physician usually as the top authority figure and the patient at the bottom of the rung, humor also serves as a leveling mechanism. It decreases the distance, and is an equalizing force.

Many of the jokes and cartoons about psychiatrists reduce this all-knowing superior being to the client's level, or at least, to a human being with a few quirks, too!

> A cartoon pictures a psychiatrist's office. The patient and psychiatrist are moving the couch across the room. The psychiatrist is saying, "Frankly, Mrs. Watson, I liked the furniture the way it was."

In the early days of social psychiatry, during the development of one community mental health center, in the attempt to move from an illness orientation to one of "health," and to foster the "blurring of roles," the staff wore ordinary street clothes rather than uniforms. The Clinical Director, however, insisted that the staff still wear name tags, which spelled out: *Jane Doe, R.N.,* and *David Brown, M.D.* The staff objected that this violated the intent of the change. The Director countered that the patients would feel more secure if they knew who the staff were. The controversy ended very suddenly when one of the day care patients appeared one morning with a name tag which read *Mary Smith, N.U.T.* The name tags went the way of the uniforms!

The need to reduce the distance between levels of staff is also facilitated through the use of humor. The jocularity, bantering, and occasional joke-telling sets a tone for a cohesiveness, a team spirit, a working together in a therapeutic atmosphere. Humor among colleagues relaxes the rigidity of the social structure without upsetting it.

When a very famous and prominent surgeon became ill and was to be admitted to the hospital as a patient, the staff of that ward became quite anxious at the thought of having to care for this authority figure. Finally, one of the nurses drew a stick figure of the surgeon "in flight" with the caption, "We've got you now!" and pinned it to his bed. When he arrived and saw the note, he burst into laughter. His subsequent sojourn in the hospital went smoothly! With one small bit of humor, the staff were able to convey their anxiety and concern and remind him that he was now in a reverse role. With his laughter, the surgeon also acknowledged his acceptance of the patient role. Within minutes an important message was conveyed that might have taken days and much emotional energy to accomplish otherwise.

Coping with Social Conflict

Rules about social conduct and behavior are carefully defined within our society: how we cover our bodies, how and where we perform bodily functions, taboos about touching our bodies, and conventions about the use of certain words in our conversations. Within the health-illness setting, under the "medical aegis," many of these rules are violated or ignored.

The patient is put to bed in the middle of the day, in an atmosphere similar to Grand Central Station, where all manner of strange persons view his nakedness, and prod and poke at him. The most intimate details are discussed within hearing distance of any number of strangers, including the stranger in the next bed. However, the rules of the game are that no one (either patient or professional) is to show embarrassment. Rather, each is expected to assume an air of detachment and nonchalance. Humor provides a very convenient means for neutralizing these emotionally tinged areas and ensuring that quality of casualness. Jokes about exposure, bedpans, enemas, bathrooms, etc. abound. The story is told in a number of ways of the succession of males in white, including the painter, who lifts the sheet to examine the female patient. One patient, who had been systematically exposed, quipped, "I have never felt so naked in my life!"

Performing bodily functions has always been a very private affair in our culture. Whether our bowels moved yesterday is not considered in the same category as the weather as a topic of general conversation (with the exception of TV commercials which discuss "irregularity" with regularity!). Yet, within the hospital or health setting, we are asked to perform on command when specimens are needed; the bedridden patient must be helped and the subject becomes one of normal everyday conversation. On an ambulatory care ward, a patient had signed out to go to the dining room and left a message on the sign board:

> Happy is the patient in the P.M.
> who has had a B.M. in the A.M.

The story is also told of the nurse who went to work as a waitress. When questioned about the change, she said, "See all those people eating out there? Well, tomorrow, I won't have to worry about whether their bowels moved or not!"

Words are coined by patients to neutralize this subject also. "The Throne" is a common expression for the bedpan while "the vase" is used for the urinal. The uninitiated who are not tuned in to these euphemisms can create situational humor.

> A young student nurse, unaware of the term used for the urinal, hesitated, when asked by a patient for a "vase." She looked around and finally asked, "Well, how big is your bouquet?"

Another of the conflicts which face both patients and personnel is in the area of the physical examination, particularly of the genital-rectal area. For the female, the pelvic examination is a routine gynecological and obstetrical procedure. Yet it is the "ultimate invasion of privacy that a conscious patient experiences."[10] The discomfort and distaste with which the patient views this procedure has nothing to do with prospect of pain, but rather with the social attitudes toward touching another's genital and rectal areas. Joan Emerson found in her study that it was usually the staff (most often the male doctor) who initiated the joking around the pelvic examination. It seems to be "an institutionalized way the staff coax the patients to put up with affronts to their dignity."[11] Patients initiate joking more often with the nurses rather than with the male doctors.

With the advent of the expanded role of the nurse and primary care responsibilities, the nurse is now also performing complete physical examinations. This often includes male patients as well as female. Traditionally, procedures related to the genital-urinary-rectal area for male patients have been delegated to the male nurses or orderlies. What this new role will do to the relationship to humor is not known, but there has always been a high incidence of joking behavior between male patients and female staff. Emerson found this humor combination considerably higher than any other combination.

Not only is teasing and joking closely related to flirting and what flirtation can lead to, but in a provocative situation like the health setting where male-female roles are distorted and many of the social rules are suspended, there are confusion and conflict as to appropriate behavior. Many male patients who are placed in this dependent position, who feel powerless, whose body image and masculinity have been threatened, typically respond with sexually oriented joking. This type of humor, in which the patient is relating to the nurse as a man to a woman rather than a patient to an authority figure, asserts his masculinity. If he also makes the nurse embarrassed and uncomfortable, he asserts his superiority over the situation.

Male patients often tell risqué jokes or tease the nurse about "back rubs" and "finishing the bath." A young male patient who had received only a piece of squash for lunch was teased for days by his roommate (in the presence of the nurse) that he had been so excited by the "sweet young student nurse" that he "couldn't even order lunch."

The nurse, who may be reacting as a female and does not recognize the patient's behavior as defensive and useful to him at this point, may begin to wonder what she has done to encourage this behavior, and become defensive herself. If, however, she recognizes the need behind the humor and responds with banter, she can use this as a cue to other impending threats to his ego.

Promoting Group Cohesion and Social Control

Promoting group solidarity is a well-known function of humor. Laughter brings people close together. To share common experiences through jocular talk forms a bond and a cohesiveness. Jocular talk differs from a joke in that the humor depends on a knowledge of the actual situation or events and a shared experience. "It unites the group by allowing it to reinterpret together an experience that previously was individual to each."[12] Within the hospital setting, jokes about the noise and activity ("I'll be glad to get home to get some rest"), poor food, getting shot "like a pin cushion," and nurses who wake you up to give you sleeping pills are common. The humorous note reduces the tension, but also serves to socialize patients into the hospital society. Through making light of this culture with all its conflicts, patients adjust to it and cope with it. Their cohesion not only reinforces the hospital structure, but through the humor teaches other patients how to adapt to it.

The professionals also have their own set of jokes and joking content which provides for group solidarity and adaptation into a profession and within an establishment in which the same social conflicts are present. There are the "in" jokes which only the "in" group understands, but which facilitates the group process and the welding of that group.

There is banter, "Do I have to work with you, again?" or the adoption of names like "The Sheik" for the surgeon who wears that particular head covering. Student nurses frequently utilize new professional terminology or jargon in their joking with each other. During a practice session in a classroom on the use of the otoscope, the student nurse who had just had a clinical experience in Obstetrics quipped to the other student who was examining her ear, "How many fingers?"

PSYCHOLOGICAL FUNCTIONS

In addition to — or concomitant with — all the social conflicts, the patient also faces many intrapsychic stresses and conflicts when illness strikes, hospitalization occurs, and disability and death threaten. Humor often is a coping mechanism. It relieves anxiety and tension, serves as an outlet for hostility and anger, provides an escape from reality, and lightens the heaviness related to permanent physical damage and death.

Relief of Anxiety, Stress and Tension

Anxiety is, perhaps, one of the most common sources of discomfort which prompts the use of humor. The "nervous giggle" is almost a physiological response for some persons. Some authors claim that anxiety is the basic emotion underlying all expressions of humor. This is a matter for debate. There is no doubt that it is inherent in many situations, and in some situations it is the prevailing or predominant theme.

If we look carefully at the current jokes, the humorous greeting cards, we can detect the anxieties of the times. Approaching middle-age (one never admits that he is already there!) is one of these. A belated birthday card sent to a friend of mine reads: "I'm sorry this card is so late, but I wasn't sure you wanted to be reminded that it was your birthday. Next year, let me know, would you rather be old or forgotten?"

The number of humorous get-well cards as well as jokes and cartoons about illnesses, hospitals, doctors, psychiatrists, and nurses attest also to this area as one of the anxieties of our society.

A cartoon shows a hospital room with two patients in bed. One is saying to the other, 'Look, you phone down to the desk and ask about my condition, and I'll phone down and ask about you.'

A get-well card says, 'Remember, it's okay to let your doctor joke with you a little...but, don't let him needle you!'

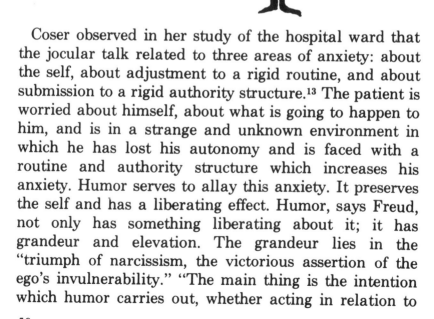

Coser observed in her study of the hospital ward that the jocular talk related to three areas of anxiety: about the self, about adjustment to a rigid routine, and about submission to a rigid authority structure.[13] The patient is worried about himself, about what is going to happen to him, and is in a strange and unknown environment in which he has lost his autonomy and is faced with a routine and authority structure which increases his anxiety. Humor serves to allay this anxiety. It preserves the self and has a liberating effect. Humor, says Freud, not only has something liberating about it; it has grandeur and elevation. The grandeur lies in the "triumph of narcissism, the victorious assertion of the ego's invulnerability." "The main thing is the intention which humor carries out, whether acting in relation to the self or other people." It means, "Look! Here is the world, which seems so dangerous! It is nothing but a game for children — just worth making a jest about."[14]

The anxiety about the seriousness of his illness, the procedures he must undergo, the loss of body parts, changes in body image, permanent disabilities like loss of hearing and blindness, prospects of pain and suffering, and threats of impending death are all areas which precipitate the use of humor.

Students, in the health professions in their initial reactions to the "reality shocks" of the health settings also utilize humor to relieve the anxiety and stress. James Thurber once said: "Humor is often emotional chaos remembered in tranquility."

In areas like intensive care units, coronary care units, emergency rooms, and operating rooms where the situation is tense, the anxiety for both patients and staff is high, and the possibility of death is a threat, there is often a great deal of joking and humor.

The level of jocular talk in the operating room by staff often indicates the level of tension. New students sometimes react negatively, depending on their own level of anxiety, particularly if the humor becomes too macabre or risqué.

When anxiety or tension is too high, humor may fall flat. According to Freud, enjoyment of the comic cannot emerge unless there is a "release of distressing effects."[15] If there is pain or anxiety and the person is himself a victim, all his energy is needed for warding off the danger and the comic effect is lost. Anxiety must be somewhat controlled before reference to it may be enjoyed in the comic or humorous situation.

Jacob Levine, in a study based on this theory, found that a joke seems funny only if it arouses anxiety and at the same time relieves it.[16] There are three types of reactions to a joke or humorous happening, he says: If it evokes no anxiety, the listener will be indifferent to the joke; if it evokes anxiety and immediately dispels it, he will find it funny; if it arouses anxiety without dissipating it, he will react with disgust, shame, embarrassment or horror.

When an elderly, dying patient moaned in pain, "Oh God, dear God," an intern stepped behind a screen and said, "This is God. What do you want?" Everyone on the ward reacted with disgust rather than laughter, because for them the anxiety was not relieved, although for the intern it was an unfortunate attempt to relieve his feelings of helplessness in the situation.

Release of Hostility and Anger

The use of humor to express feelings of anger, hostility, and frustration is perhaps one of the most difficult areas for people to accept; yet this is by far one of the most constructive functions of humor.

The outward expression of anger and aggression in our society is generally frowned upon and creates almost as much conflict in our society as sex! But to express hostility through joking is socially acceptable because the target of the hostility can laugh with you. It is a face-saving device. Yet he gets the point. Studies have shown that the enjoyment of aggressive or hostile humor has led to a decrease in hostile feelings. The release of anger in a witty way may do much to prevent the outbreak of hostility or the bottling up of frustration. Within the hospital society there are many sources of anger and frustration. As in society in general, the outward expression of these is usually looked upon with disfavor.

> The physician had ordered all stools to be saved on a patient who had been admitted for tests and observation. The nursing staff had disposed of those which were filled with barium and enema returns as not valuable. The doctor, however, quite upset at this decision, rewrote the order to read: "Save everything that emits from the anal canal." The staff not only proceeded to send buckets of enema returns to the lab, but also took a large plastic bag

used for linen, filled it with air, and labeled it "fresh flatus."

The rigidity of the hospital routines and their dehumanizing elements often leaves the patient feeling angry and frustrated. To be openly hostile is contrary to the "good" patient role and might alienate the staff upon whom he relies for care. Therefore, the jocular gripe or joke provides an outlet and performs both the function of complaint and joke. The humor is a safety valve. Comments like "Where else can you get ice water at 5:30 a.m.?" are such evidences of frustration. The patient's anger at his own illness is also often revealed and dissipated through the use of humor. One patient referred to his colostomy as "Old Stinky."

The dehumanizing quality of all the new medical technologies resulted in another patient describing himself as "an extension of the machine." Another patient, alone in an isolation room, put a sign on her door. "If you're afraid of the bugs, at least knock when you go by!"

William Fry describes the relationship between humor, play, and fighting, which, he says, may explain the frequent association of aggression and hostility with humor.[17]

Children and animals "horse around," wrestle playfully, slap and push and nip at each other, yet never really hurt each other. It is difficult sometimes to distinguish between play and fighting and where one stops and the other begins. The participants, however, determine that they are playing, not fighting, and therefore, there must be meta-communications, cues, messages which say: "This slap is in fun — not in anger." Therefore, there is a "play frame" which says, "This is play — it is not real," although the slap itself is real. The same kind of meta-communication occurs in humor and sets a joke frame. It says, "This is a joke — it is not for real." "It is just play." We say, "Have you heard this one?" Thus we set the stage for the punch line, to which the surprised listener reacts with laughter. In burlesque, it is called the "sock line."

The word *punch* probably originated from Punchinello (a medieval Italian comedy figure), and the Punch and Judy shows, and *Punch*, the English humorous weekly. All derive from the Italian word, *polcino*, for chicken. As Fry says, the cocky rooster, an honored figure in the tradition of comedy, reveals some truths about ourselves as represented by life in a barnyard!

There is a pecking order to joke telling. The joke teller is the dominant one; the joke is his weapon; his laughter is the sign of victory. The audience is submissive; their laughter is the sign of their acceptance of defeat. "I give up," they say. Then the pecking order gets reversed. "Hey, I've got one!" There are joke orgies in which everyone gets a chance to "punch" it to the others.

Certain figures of speech in our language reveal this aggressive component: "a disarming smile," "a winning smile," "weak with laughter," "a triumphant laugh," "Smile when you say that," and so on.

Many authors, as I have indicated before, see humor as a way to reduce aggression in our society to a tolerable level. Certainly, both patients and staff can use humor effectively to release bottled-up frustrations and hostility.

Denial of Reality

Many instances of humor serve to deny or avoid feelings which are too painful or distressful. The "cut-up" very often falls into this category. He does not stop long enough to allow himself to feel. In many instances, when the stress is too great, this mechanism is one of self-preservation until the person is able emotionally to deal with it.

Lord Byron once wrote:
"And if I laugh at any mortal thing,
'Tis that I may not weep."

Freud has said that in humor the ego refuses to be distressed by reality, or to let itself suffer. In fact, these traumas are occasions for it to gain pleasure.

When a group of young people were involved in a near fatal accident, the driver of the car called home to tell her parents. The mother, hearing laughter in the background, asked her daughter how they could laugh! She said, "Mother, if we didn't laugh, we couldn't stand all this!" One of the others, who had been asleep in the back seat of the car, quipped, "First accident I've ever been in, and I had to sleep through it!"

Many patients use humor to deny the seriousness of their illness. The humorous get-well cards on the market today may be an indication of a denial of these feelings, also. According to Norris it is a "cover it up with a laugh" or an expression of helplessness even though the person is concerned about the patient. It may be sending a message which says "I hope you are not really ill; therefore, this lighthearted card is appropriate — I hope, I hope, I hope."[18]

Coping with Disabilities and Death

The hospital is a place where many of the problems from which others in society attempt to insulate themselves must be faced by both patients and staff. Death is one of these. Humor is a technique used to neutralize this emotionally charged event.

The type of humor often used in tragic situations is described as grim humor or gallows humor from Freud's famous story of the rogue who was being led to the gallows. It was a Monday and the condemned man remarked "Well, this week's beginning nicely."[19] Although pity is initiated for the condemned man, his stoic jibe saves the person listening the expenditure of energy needed to suppress the painful emotion of pity and instead he laughs. In other words, the rogue says: "Don't pity me, laugh with me."

This bravado in the face of death was also described in the report by Renee Fox in which, as a sociologist, she discussed what happened on a small experimental metabolic ward. Because of the gravity of the diseases the physicians had to deal with, the constant possibilities of failure and death, the problems of uncertainty, and the trial-and-error nature of coping with these uncertainties, a highly patterned and intricate form of humor evolved. As one physician said, "Our humor is a kind of protective device. If we were to talk seriously all the time and act like a bunch of Sir Galahads or something, we just couldn't take all this."[20]

The type of joking seen in this group is so characteristic of physicians, Fox says, that it is generally referred to as "Medical Humor." In the earliest years of their medical training, physicians learn that an effective and appropriate way to handle their reactions to death and other stressful or emotionally provocative professional situations is to joke with their colleagues about them in a look-it-in-the-face-and-laugh manner.

The patients in this setting also used humor as a way of coping with their stresses, but, as Emerson found in her study, rarely did this humor cross the status lines. Staff joked among themselves, but they rarely joked with patients or visitors. Sometimes, the patient himself initiated the humor: "How's my blood pressure? Do you think I'll live?"

> The doctor was visiting his 90-year-old patient. She asked him, "Do you think I'll get well?" He answered

sadly, "I hope so — but we doctors aren't magicians. We can't make our patients younger." Her eyes twinkled. "But Doctor," she said, "I don't want you to make me younger. I want you to help me get older."[21]

However, the studies by Fox and Emerson were done in 1959 and 1962. In the past several years, with the concern for the dying patient and the education of the professional toward openness and understanding and intervention in the grieving process, the communication patterns have changed. It is possible that the use of humor is changing also.

Recently, a patient recovering from heart surgery commented, "When you wake up you're convinced you didn't make it, but you're not sure you made heaven either!"

Mikes points out that death is a part of human life and man has joked about death ever since he was born.[22] The literature is full of funny deaths and funerals. Laughing at death, he says, gives triple pleasure: the pleasure of the joke itself, the malicious joy of laughing at death's expense, and the pleasure of taming death and fraternizing with him.

Because this end of the continuum, the dealing with tragedy through humor, is one which raises the most questions and around which one must look most closely at whose needs are being met, the comparison of gallows humor and its relation to the black humor of fiction and to "medical humor" will be discussed in the next chapter.

That even the dying patient can utilize humor is shown by this excerpt from a letter written by a patient dying from cancer, just two weeks before her death.

> I think it is time we let down our hair and told the truth. We have the urge to rush into print all right, but we who are dying of cancer are not martyrs or saints or holy folk. Frankly, if the truth were told we embarrass our friends and we often bore them!...
>
> I'm still angry about it all, for I think no one has ever loved living more or had more fun doing it than I, and I

want it to go on and on. But if I can't, then I must be truthful and say there are a few advantages in living only half a lifetime. Besides the end of good, death also means the end of tribulations — no more holding in the stomach, no more P.T.A., no more putting up the hair in pincurls, no more cub scouts, no more growing old.[23]

SUMMARY

We have described some general purposes and uses for humor within the health setting. In the next chapters we will discuss the use of the gallows type humor by staff as well as patient, use of humor in psychiatry and psychotherapy, and the use of humor in education, particularly the education of the health professional.

Humor can heal! Learning how to use it effectively is necessary.

REFERENCES

1. Coser RL: Some social functions of laughter: a study of humor in a hospital setting. *In* Skipper JK, Leonard RC (eds): *Social Interaction and Patient Care.* Philadelphia, JB Lippincott, 1965, pp 292-306.
2. Fox RC: *Experiment Perilous.* Glencoe, Ill, The Free Press, 1959.
3. Emerson JP: *Humor in Hospital Setting,* 1963.
4. Robinson VM: Humor in nursing. *In* Carlson C (ed): *Behavioral Concepts and Nursing Intervention.* Philadelphia, JB Lippincott, 1970, pp 129-51. (This is the initial study of humor by this author, some of which is incorporated into this chapter.)
5. Emerson, *Humor in Hospital Setting,* pp 332-334.
6. Fry, *Sweet Madness,* p 67.
7. Emerson, *Humor in Hospital Setting,* p 47.
8. Coser, *Social Functions of Laughter,* p 293.
9. *Ibid,* p 304.
10. Emerson, *Humor in Hospital Setting,* p 167.
11. *Ibid,* p 212.
12. Coser, *Social Functions of Laughter,* p 301.
13. *Ibid,* p 295.
14. Freud, *Humor,* p 166.
15. Freud, *Jokes,* p 228.
16. Levine J: Responses to humor. *Scientific American* 194:31-35, 1950.
17. Fry, *Sweet Madness,* pp 101-115.
18. Norris C: Greetings from the lonely crowd. *Nursing Forum* 1:73-82, 1961-62.
19. Freud, *Humor,* p 161; and *Jokes,* p 229.
20. Fox, *Experiment,* p 81.
21. Robinson R; More candles for her cake. *RN* 27:57, August 1964.
22. Mikes, *Laughing Matter,* p 40.
23. Beland IL: *Clinical Nursing.* New York: The Macmillan Co, 1965, pp 89-91.

"medical" humor as g^allows humor

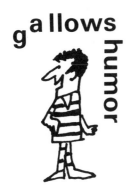

Man alone suffers so excruciatingly in the world that he was compelled to invent laughter.

NIETZSCHE

We have identified the "need" continuum in regard to humor as ranging essentially from simple pleasure to tragedy. We have also established, however, that the need for humor is a very individual phenomenon. How, then, do the two participants, health-care-giver and health-care-receiver, utilize this humor? Is it a mutual exchange or is it mutually exclusive? At the pleasure end, if the pleasantry, for example, involves only staff who are ignoring the patient, humor can be disconcerting for the patient. However, at the other end of the continuum, if the health professional is attempting to meet his own anxieties about the tragedy which is occurring and if his style of humor does not help the patient who is distressed from a different vantage point (it is happening to him!), humor can be more than simply disconcerting!

Since the style of humor at this end of the continuum is often one of satire or a grim, gallows type of humor, very similar to the black humor style of fiction, we need to compare the styles and techniques, and to explore this

59

whole area of the relationship between laughter and tears, comedy and tragedy, and the "gallows" humor to which "medical" humor has been likened.

COMEDY VERSUS TRAGEDY

This theme or thread of the relationship of humor and laughter with tragedy and tears, the assumption that we laugh so that we may not cry (although sometimes we laugh so hard we *do* cry!), has permeated a majority of the writings on humor. The relationship is not clearly understood, but that the relationship exists is firmly acknowledged. "Man is the only animal that laughs and weeps" says William Hazlitt, "To explain the nature of laughter and tears is to account for the condition of human life."[1]

Koestler places comedy on a continuum with tragedy, and describes laughter and tears as similar "luxury reflexes," which seem to have no apparent biological purposes but provide a similar obvious relief.[2]

Bonamy Dobree distinguishes between three kinds of comedy: "critical" comedy, "free" comedy, and a third comedy which he calls "great" comedy. This comedy is perilously near tragedy and deals with the disillusion of mankind, the failures of men to realize their most passionate desires. This comedy makes daily life livable, he says:

> ... [it] gives us courage to face life without any standpoint, we need not view it critically or feel heroically. We need only to feel humanly, for comedy shows us life not at such a distance that we cannot but regard it coldly, but only so far as we may bring to it a ready sympathy freed from terror or too overwhelming a measure of pity.[3]

This acceptance of "living" is similar in many ways to the acceptance of "death and dying." Kubler-Ross and others have spoken to the need to accept human finiteness and the inevitability of one's own death before the professional can be therapeutic with the dying patient. So, also, the acceptance of human imperfection — and one's own humanness — through comedy and humor manages to assist the individual with the realities of life and living. Humor assists in the retention of hope. If we can joke, things cannot possibly be so bad!

The concept of humor and laughter as a relief from and a way of coping with the realities of life and of dying is an important consideration. Even the "harmless" and "empty" jokes and those of "sheer delight" seem to be a way to avoid emotion, to relieve us of the burdens of reality. When we are immersed in a joke and in the throes of laughter, for that moment, at least, all other thoughts are forgotten. In the life-and-death arena of health and illness, where tragedy and living are highlighted, the role that humor may play in acceptance of both could be vital.

GALLOWS HUMOR

Freud's basic concept that joking relieves repressed impulses and anxieties, and that laughter converts the unpleasant feelings to pleasant ones, underlies the theory of "gallows humor." This gallows humor, a grim, macabre humor, a bravado in the face of death, is a type of humor which is typically seen when individuals or groups are faced with considerable stress and precarious or dangerous situations, such as war, on battlefields, in oppressed countries, in concentration camps, and in life-and-death struggles within hospitals.

Obrdlik describes it as a social phenomenon which has a definite purpose, that is, to ridicule with irony, invectives, and sarcasm in order to become a means of an effective social control. It provides a psychological escape and strengthens the morale of the group at the same time that it undermines the morale of the oppressors.

During the early days of the Nazi movement before the actual invasion of Czechoslovakia, the ridiculing of the Nazi leaders and their regime through jokes and anecdotes was a lighthearted bravado and defiance which gave the people a feeling of security. Although at the point of invasion when the Czech nation was crushed and bleeding, humor temporarily disappeared, it was soon heard again, but more biting, with more irony, and directed at the Czech "traitors" as well.

Obrdlik said,

> People who live in absolute uncertainty of their lives and property find a refuge in inventing, repeating and spreading through the channels of whispering counter-propaganda, anecdotes and jokes about their oppressors...they have to strengthen their hope because otherwise they could not bear the strains to which their nerves are exposed.[4]

Some of the stories that made the rounds were:

> Do you know why Hitler has not yet invaded England? Because the German officers could not manage to learn in time all English irregular verbs.

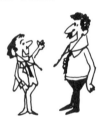

> An old man walking up the street, speaking aloud, said: "Adolf Hitler is the greatest leader.... I would rather work for ten Germans than one Czech." When the Gestapo agent asked what was his occupation, this Czech admirer of Nazism reluctantly confessed that he was a gravedigger.[5]

Obrdlik felt that what is true for individuals is also true for whole nations, namely:

> ...that the purest type of ironical humor is born out of sad experiences accompanied by grief and sorrow. It is spontaneous and deep felt — the very necessity of life which it helps to preserve.[6]

This type of humor was also seen on the battlefield, by the men fighting the wars. During World War II, the Bill Mauldin cartoons and jokes were typical. Willie and his buddy are in a foxhole amidst rubble with bullets flying overhead and he says: "I feel like a fugitive from the law of averages." In another cartoon, the chaplain has been conducting services in the foxhole and he ends with "...forever, Amen. Hit the dirt!"[7] During the Vietnam War, Mauldin produced a cartoon, showing a GI coming through the jungle. A signpost on which Indochina is crossed out and Vietnam is added is attached to a tree. Propped against that tree is a skeleton with a grinning skull clothed in the uniform of a French soldier. The GI is saying, "What's so funny, Monsieur? I'm only trying to find my way."[8]

BLACK HUMOR OF FICTION

Black humor (not to be confused with Afro-American humor) has been the subject of much controversy. It has been described as a humor of "grotesque exaggeration, extravagance, sexuality and violence"[9] and seen as typical of American humor from its beginnings; it will continue to express the American character in the future. Max Schulz calls it an absurdity in existentialist fiction, a divergence from traditional comedy and satire, which "condemns man to a dying world."[10] Bruce Jay Friedman who coined the term *black humor* suggests that the "chord of absurdity" was struck merely by recording the events of the present age! The satirist had to go beyond satire because his ground had been usurped by the newspaper reporter. Finally, black humor has been defined as a "bitter emphasis on the absurd that makes us laugh so that we will not cry."[11] Joseph Heller, who wrote the classic *Catch-22*, once said that he wanted people to laugh and then look back in horror at what they were laughing at.

When the world could no longer avoid or deny the emotionality of the grim prospects of death, of racial tensions, threats to establishments and changing sexual mores, and when the empty, bland, harmless humor of the Fifties no longer sufficed, the grotesque absurdist fiction of black humor arose. It was a move to the opposite extreme: "making fun of," in the most grotesque, macabre manners, those very things which frightened and disturbed society. It seemed to be almost an attempt to "shock" ourselves out of the horror and anxiety. If we shout the four-letter words often enough, detail the most intimate sexual experience often enough, revel in the most macabre aspects of illness and death often enough, relate the lurid aspects of war and riot and killings often enough, soon they become commonplace, meaningless and emotionless!

In black humor, death and illness and disease and bodily injury are dealt with in a similar, macabre way although through the eyes of the lay person rather than the professional. In the two classics, *Catch-22* and *One Flew Over the Cuckoo's Nest,* the whole medical system is satirized. From the perspective of the patient, fears, horrors, and anxieties about illness and death are grotesquely revealed as well as the incompetencies of the health professionals and the corruptness and dehumanizing quality of the health system.

Catch-22 revolves around the fear of death felt by the chief character, Yossarian, and his attempts to avoid the bombing missions and stay alive.

> Yossarian was a lead bombardier who had been demoted because he no longer gave a damn whether he missed or not. He had decided to live forever or die in the attempt and his only mission each time he went up was to come down alive.[12]

Yossarian's thoughts about death are thrust at the reader again and again.

> ...a placid blue sea...that could gulp down a person with a cramp in the twinkling of an eye and ship him back to shore three days later, all charges paid, bloated, blue and putrescent, water draining out through both cold nostrils.[13]
>
> People knew a lot more about dying inside the hospital

and made a much neater, more orderly job of it. They couldn't dominate Death inside the hospital, but they certainly made her behave. They had taught her manners.... There was none of that crude, ugly ostentation about dying that was so common outside the hospital.... People didn't stick their heads into ovens with the gas on, jump in front of subway trains or come plummeting like dead weights out of hotel windows with a whoosh! Accelerating at the rate of thirty-two feet per second to land with a hideous plop! on the sidewalk and die disgustingly there in public like an alpaca sack full of hairy strawberry ice cream, bleeding, pink toes awry.[14]

The whole crazy medical system to which Yossarian looks for help by his frequent visits to the hospital to avoid flying is also satirized. The physician, Doc Daneeka, is an absurd figure who —

...brooded over his health continually and went almost daily to the medical tent to have his temperature taken by one of the two enlisted men there who ran things for him practically on their own, and ran it so efficiently that he was left with little else to do but sit in the sunlight with his stuffed nose and wonder what other people were so worried about.[15]

The two enlisted men, Gus and Wes,

...succeeded in elevating medicine to exact science. All men...with temperatures above 102° were rushed to the hospital. All those except Yossarian...with temperatures below 102° had their gums and toes painted with Gentian Violet solution and were given a laxative to throw away into the bushes.[16]

Of course, the "soldier in white, who could not have been any sicker without being dead," is the epitome of the grotesque. Encased from head to toe in plaster and gauze with only an empty dark hole over his mouth, and all four limbs hoisted in the air by cable and weights, he is fed by his own wastes.

A silent zinc pipe rose from the cement on his groin and was coupled to a slim rubber hose that carried waste from his kidneys and dripped it efficiently into a clear, stoppered jar on the floor. When the jar was full, the jar feeding his elbow was empty; and the two were simply switched so that stuff could drip into him.[17]

The "mechanical encrusted on the living" is vividly displayed in the reaction to the soldier who was "more like a stuffed and sterilized mummy." "Nurse Duckett and Nurse Cramer kept him spic and span." They brushed his bandages with a whiskbroom, scrubbed the casts, polished the pipes and glass jars. "They were proud of their homework." Yossarian and the other patients wonder if he can hear; if he's breathing if it never moves; and, if it's a he! Yossarian finally asks the nurse, "How the hell do you know he's even in there?"

In Kesey's *One Flew Over the Cuckoo's Nest*, the psychiatric hospital is satirized in all its bizarreness, portraying the often-held theme that the society within the hospital is "kookier" than that outside its walls, and that the so-called "therapeutic" measures only tend to reinforce the problems with which the patient enters the hospital. The big nurse, the impotent psychiatrist, and the sadistic attendants are the epitomes of all the patients' worst fears. McMurphy tries to bring some reason and normalcy into the system and we revel in all his rebellious escapades and antics. Humor and laughter is the key to the changes which he creates. He finds the patients are "scared to open up and laugh."

> You know, that's the first thing that got me about this place, that there wasn't anybody laughing. I haven't heard a real laugh since I came through the door, do you know that? Man, when you lose your laugh, you lose your footing. A man go around letten a woman whup him down till he can't laugh anymore, and he loses one of the biggest edges he's got on his side.[18]

The change to the ability to use laughter is revealed in the patients' managing the uncomfortable embarrassing situation of being sprayed for lice after their return from their boat trip.

> We lined up nude against the tile, and here one black boy came, a black plastic tube in his hand, squirting a stinking

salve thick and sticky as egg white. In the hair first, then turn around an' bend over an' spread your cheeks!

The guys complained and kidded and joked about it, trying not to look at one another or those floating slate masks working down the line behind the tubes, like nightmare faces in negative, sighting down soft, squeezy nightmare gunbarrels. They kidded the black boys by saying things like "Hey, Washington, what do you fellas do for fun the other sixteen hours?" "Hey, Williams, can you tell me what I had for breakfast?"

Everybody laughed. The black boys clenched their jaws and didn't answer; this wasn't the way things used to be before that damned redhead came around.

When Fredrickson spread his cheeks there was such a sound I thought the last black boy'd be blown clear off his feet. "Hark!" Harding said, cupping his hand to his ear. "The lovely voice of an angel."[19]

The laughing and obscene comments served the patients' needs for covering up their embarrassment and humiliation although the attendants did not find it funny!

Sex is the area, perhaps, which has gained the black humorists the most notoriety. The new morality has made this unspeakable area a more open one. The black humorists, in fact, have not only opened the door, but have thrown away the key and thrown up all the blinds. *Catch-22's* men are as obsessed with sex as they are with dying: Nately's whore, Luciana, the maid in the lime panties, Nurse Duckett, and Hungry Joe's photography.

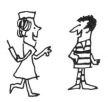

In *One Flew Over the Cuckoo's Nest,* McMurphy's record, Big Nurse's Needs, bringing in the prostitutes for the party, and Billy's virgin attempts are vividly portrayed.

PATIENTS' USE OF GALLOWS HUMOR IN THE REAL SETTING

Within the real hospital setting, patients have been observed using similar gallows type humor to cope with embarrassing intimate procedures and stressful situations.

During the second World War, on a ward of returned combat soldiers who were not only blind but had a limb or perhaps two missing, the use of humor was observed by this author as a frequent form of expression by the men. Many of the patients were fitted with artificial eyes which had to be removed and the eye socket cleaned several times a day during the adjustment period. The workmanship was so fine that it was often difficult for the nurse to tell the difference and would have to ask the patient. Frequently, he would point to the wrong one or squeeze the eye so that it dropped out and laugh hilariously at the nurse's shock and dismay. When patients walking down the hall on the center rubber runner, which was their guide, bumped into each other or into staff, the common response was, "What's the matter with you? Got eye trouble?"

In the experimental metabolic ward studied by Renee Fox, the use of humor was one of the ways patients came to terms with the problems and stresses they shared. They wrote medical documents satirizing a "case history" and a "report of death" with such statements as, "He died 'cause he was too damn lazy to live." Much of the joking revolved around the way they were subject to the medical program.

> I think the reason I'm so fouled up is because of all the gooey stuff they're always sticking in my veins. My veins must be coated an inch thick with all that sticky albumin and resin. What I need is an I.V. of Sani-Flush.[20]

They designed a coat of arms for the ward: two criss-crossed hypodermic needles, with a drop of blood suspended from the tip of each.

Finally, there were "death" jokes. "I sure came close to the pearly gates, all right! I knocked on them, but Saint Peter told me to get the hell out!" They played at summoning up spirits who came back to haunt those still alive. A patient, reacting to a group of doctors discussing his case at his bedside, joked, "You fellows better get it together quick...can't you see I'm dying?"

"MEDICAL" HUMOR

Similarly, the hospital and the health professionals in it must deal with these problems and fears, the ultimate being death with all the degrees and potentialities of that, from minor illness to critical illness to disability and disfigurement. The handling of the body and all the intimate procedures which have sexual implications is another area of conflict in our society.

The type of laughing-at-death gallows humor which Renee Fox called typical "medical" humor has been used by all health professionals in adjusting to the "reality shocks" of their chosen occupations.

Student nurses and medical students give fond names to cadavers, either human or animal, they use to study anatomy and physiology. A favorite jingle when tuberculosis sanitariums still flourished was:

> T.B. or not T.B.,
> That is congestion,
> Consumption be done about it?
> Of corpse! Of corpse!

Death and the procedure for preparing the body for the morgue often provoke a "laughing at death" approach. On one occasion, when an old gentleman had died, the two student nurses who were on duty that night, in the absence of the orderly, prepared the body for the morgue. They straightened the limbs and gently but securely tied them with gauze bandages. Then, discovering that the "sexual appendage" was erect, gaily decorated it with a huge gauze bow, brightly dotted with red and blue ink.

The frequent association of food to blood and viscera is common:

> Liver again! Pathology must have had an oversupply this week!

In the operating room and emergency room, where tension is the highest, humor becomes almost a standard pattern of interaction, from simple, jocular talk to macabre, risqué joking.

> Two students were observing surgery for the first time. The shorter one was complaining she couldn't see. The tall one quipped, "Be glad you're not tall. You have a longer way to fall when you faint!"

> During an operation, the assisting doctor told a joke: "Do you know what happened to the nurse who swallowed a razor blade? She performed a tonsillectomy, a hysterectomy, and circumcised an intern."

Renee Fox describes the form of "gallows humor" which the physicians used on the experimental metabolic ward she studied. They joked about the uncertainties, their inability to "cure" patients and some of the impending deaths; they made bets about the unknown. This freeing of tension helped them to come to terms with their situation in a useful and professionally acceptable way.

> Dr. D.: Mr. Goss is still alive.
> Dr. S.: Is he putting out urine?
> Dr. D.: No.
> Dr. E.: Is he having hemodialysis?
> Dr. D.: No.
> Dr. C.: Then how is he alive? (laughter)[21]
> Dr. C.: I'll give you 10 to 1 that Mr. Green had Addison's disease.
> Dr. D.: I won't take it...[22]

A recent book coauthored by Renee Fox on organ transplants and dialysis reinforces again the physician's use of humor as a means for coping with the uncertainty and scientific inadequacies.

GALLOWS HUMOR: WHOSE NEEDS ARE BEING MET?

The significant consideration at this point must be whether or not the gallows type of humor used by patients and by staff with their peers is appropriate to be cultivated by staff to use in interaction with patients. Sociologist Coser has suggested that humor across status lines may well take other forms and have other functions than humor among status equals. Obrdlik, in discussing the positive effect of gallows humor, also speaks to the negative effect, a disintegrating influence among those against whom it is directed, and undermining of morale. "The black humorist," Hamlin Hill contends, "does not seek the sympathy or alliance of his audience, but deliberately insults and alienates it."[23] It becomes a moot question then, since gallows humor appears to relieve one's own anxiety, not necessarily those of others, particularly when the other may be the object of the tragedy.

The medical humor generally used by the health professional has always been to support his own needs, to relieve his own anxieties and concerns, and to avoid those aspects of tragedy which he is expected to play a large part in preventing by his skills and knowledge. The paradox is that the medical humor brings him closer to his colleagues, to share in the realization that he is not a hero, is not perfect, is still human. Yet the patient is depending upon him to prevent death, to avoid disability, and to cure his illness. He is expecting and paying for seriousness, and miracles, and godliness.

Emerson states that more watchfulness is necessary in regard to humor than in most matters because by its very nature humor is always toeing the line between divergence and defiance, tottering on the verge of going too far.

In the current TV series *M*A*S*H,* this fine line seems to be achieved. They demonstrate very clearly the staff's need for humor as a way to survive that situation, yet in no way do they put down, depreciate, or laugh at the patient in this attempt. The staff still maintains that quality of concern, of caring and competency despite their zaniness. The health professional is always in a dilemma of having to present the all-knowing, miracle-worker, god-like air which patients expect, yet underneath knowing he is as human and vulnerable as the rest.

The humor between colleagues is very often a self-depreciating one, which is acceptable within status lines, but might not be understood in the same vein by the patient. This story making the rounds some years ago may serve a an example.

> Two psychiatrists are coming down in the elevator after a day in the office. The younger psychiatrist looks weary and somber. The older psychiatrist is whistling cheerfully. The younger man looks over and says, 'How can you be so spry and cheerful after a long day of listening to patients with all their problems and troubles?' The older man shrugs his shoulders and responds, 'Who listens?'

This may tickle the fantasies of the psychiatric staff, but might be very threatening to the patient who will always wonder if *his* psychiatrist is really listening!

Much more research in this area needs to be done. It may very well be that the use of gallows humor as a technique is a limited one for use by staff with patients.

However, the value and usefulness of gallows humor for each, patient and staff, individually, as a mechanism for coping cannot be overlooked, and therefore, should not be discarded. The recognition of whose needs are being met and when and in what situation seems to be the crucial factor. The fine line or delicate balance between use by staff and use by patients must be found. There may be times when a gallows-type humor may be appropriate across status lines in the right situation and the right time.

REFERENCES

1. Hazlett W: On wit and humour. *In* Enck JJ, Forter ET, Whitley A (eds): *The Comic in Theory and Practice,* p 16.
2. Koestler, *Act of Creation,* p 31.
3. Dobree B, *Restoration Comedy,* p 205.
4. Obrdlik AJ, *Gallows Humor,* p 712.
5. *Ibid,* p 713-714.
6. *Ibid,* p 715.
7. Mauldin B: *The Brass Ring.* New York, WW Norton and Co, 1971, pp 217-219.
8. Mauldin B: *I've Decided I Want My Seat Back.* New York, Harper and Row, 1965, p 110.
9. Sklar R: Humor in America. *In* Mendel WM (ed): *A Celebration of Laughter.* Los Angeles, Mara Books, 1970, p 28.
10. Schulz MF: *Black Humor Fiction in the Sixties.* Athens, Ohio, Ohio University Press, 1973, p 7.
11. Muller WJ, Nelson BE: *Joseph Heller's Catch-22.* Monarch Notes. New York, Monarch Press, 1971, p 6.
12. Heller J: *Catch 22.* New York, Dell Publishing Co., 1955, p 30.
13. *Ibid,* p 18.
14. *Ibid,* p 170-71.
15. *Ibid,* p 33.
16. *Ibid,* p 31.
17. *Ibid,* p 10.
18. Kesey K: *One Flew Over The Cuckoo's Nest,* New York, Signet Books, 1962, pp 65-66.
19. *Ibid,* p 227.
20. Fox R, *Experiment Perilous,* p 171.
21. *Ibid,* p 78.
22. *Ibid,* p 82.
23. Hill H: Black humor and its causes and cure. *Colorado Quarterly* XVII:59, 1968.

BIBLIOGRAPHY

Boskin J: Black/Black humor: the renaissance of laughter. *In* Mendel WM (ed): *A Celebration of Laughter.* Los Angeles, Mara Books, Inc, 1970, pp 147-148.
Fox RC, Swazey JP: *The Courage to Fail.* Chicago, University of Chicago Press, 1974.
Koestler A: *The Act of Creation,* 1964.

humor 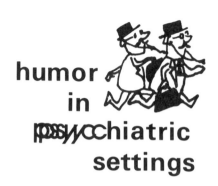 in psychiatric settings

Traditionally, we have laughed at the "crazy" behavior of the mentally ill person. Many jokes, cartoons, and comedies revolve around and mimic this abnormal behavior. The professional who works with emotionally disturbed persons often justifies his laughter as the only way he can keep his own sanity. However, traditionally, this disparaging laughter never occurs in the presence of the patient. Rather, the "seriousness" of the situation and the "mental state" of the patient have always precluded the use of humor as appropriate in the treatment or therapy of the psychiatric patient.

Most of the objections have come from classical psychoanalysts, which is all the more surprising since:

> Freud made a pioneering effort to equate maturity with humor, theorizing that both the production and appreciation of humor mirror the triumph of narcissism and the pleasure principle over an array of stressful environmental circumstances.[1]

Walter O'Connell, who apparently has spent a considerable portion of his professional life attempting experimentally to prove Freud's theory, goes on to say:

> Since a sense of humor has often been mentioned as the 'sine qua non' of the mature person, it is paradoxical that very little effort has been expended in attempts to define and measure this key concept.[2]

O'Connell based most of these studies on the differentiation between humor, wit, and resignation. Freud, he said, made sharp distinctions between these, but most subsequent investigators tended to overlook this, particularly the analysts, who examined wit rather than humor, but, unfortunately, labeled their study subject as humor. To Freud, humor is the epitome of maturity, an adaptive mechanism used by well-adjusted people, seen as an empathetic nonrepressing awareness of the "littleness of man." Freud's example of gallows humor is really dealing with death in a nonhostile way. The rogue's, "Well, this week's beginning nicely," does not offend others, and shows the ability to jest even at life's final moment of stress. Resignation shows the same nondecompensating behavior, but without the enlivening jests. The rogue is more resigned to his fate, "The world won't come to an end." Tendentious wit, on the other hand, is hostile wit, employed by less adjusted persons, and is regarded as the sudden release of hostile or sexually repressed drives, albeit in a socially acceptable way. The same rogue, according to O'Connell, using hostile wit, might have said to his fellow prisoners as he is led to the gallows, "You cats will be dancing on air soon, too."[3] Humor is an attitude; wit is a mechanism.

A search through the biographies of the giants of psychiatry shows that these men were hypersensitive to death through traumatic experiences, but later in life developed and communicated a deep empathy and humor-like approach to life's inevitabilities. In an experiment conducted with first-year medical students comparing their future speciality choices with their attitudes toward death and appreciation of humor, O'Connell found potential psychiatrists did not have this same maturity and had higher concerns about their own deaths than any other specialty area. Potential surgeons had the lowest concerns about death! There were no significant differences, however, between choice of humor, wit, or resignation as compared to nonmedical college students, implying that college students have not yet reached the level of maturity for humor, as opposed to wit. O'Connell suggests that potential psychiatrists may need education toward increased empathy and humor to make death concerns a professional asset.

The lack of focus on humor as a factor in therapy and the present controversial opinions may very well have been the result, as O'Connell indicates, of Freud concentrating on the hostile wit rather than the mature, empathetic humor.

Freud has been described as a storyteller and lover of jokes who utilized his patient's jokes and his patient's dreams, which were full of jokes and puns, in his treatment. Alfred Adler was also described as having an abundance of humor. Adlerian psychotherapy, which emphasizes encouragement as a primary technique and keeping the patient's hope elevated as one factor in this technique, suggests that humor assists in the retention of this hope.

Other analysts have suggested that eliciting from patients their favorite jokes could be useful in revealing anxiety around areas of conflict and repression. Zwerling points out that this technique may lead lightly and naturally into discussions of such areas of conflict and may be particularly useful when a light touch is needed for a tentative approach to a troubled area.[4] This technique offers insights in the same way as dreams, memories, and responses to projective techniques, but has the advantage of being more concise and pointed. However, this technique has several limitations, Zwerling says, which are valuable points to be considered. Some patients fail to have a favorite joke and some patients may resort to the latest joke they heard. The "favorite joke" may also be a learned one, that is, told with repeated success several times, so that it achieves the status of favorite joke, but does not bear any relationship to the problems of the teller. Other limitations may be that the joke may reflect the social problems of the patient's particular culture, but may not necessarily represent his specific conflict. Or a patient's neurosis may be so complex that a great variety of jokes would reflect some aspect of his personality. However, he says, this technique should be useful in any system of therapy that recognizes the personality as a unit in which every part is related to the whole.

In contrast, adding to the controversy, Morris Brody maintains that laughter is not common during the analytic hour except as a reaction to occasional wit, and, as a rule, it is the sickest type of personalities (the schizophrenic, schizoid or compulsive) who smiles or laughs during the analytic session. The analyst may call attention to his laughter, but once this happens, the patient becomes uneasy, fearing he is being laughed at or accused of having laughed at the analyst. Laughter, Brody says, is a defense best left undisturbed because the meaning of the laughter is too buried in the unconscious.[5]

Nussbaum and Michaux explain that the schizophrenic's inability to experience humor is a result of his conceptual disorganization which interferes with his "getting the point of a joke" but that the patient with an affective disorder will at least intellectually understand it. The inability of the depressed patient to react to humor may be due to a "freeze of affect," if it is certain that he has not been too preoccupied to listen to the joke and to understand it. On this assumption, then, the reaction of the depressed patient to humor could be utilized as a predictor of the course of the illness. As the depression lifts, his ability to react to humor may improve. The results of experimental study by Nussbaum and Michaux offered tentative support to this theory. They found reactive depressives responded better than psychotic depressives with grandiose guilt feelings but that in patients with schizophrenic overtones, the schizophrenic ideation increased.[6]

In a situation observed by this author, a patient who became depressed following gallbladder surgery demonstrated this increased response to humor as her depression lifted. It had been noted, however, that the patient had often used humor as her pattern of interaction prior to surgery. The nursing staff in their plan for nursing care utilized humor as an approach to intervening in the depressive reaction with subsequent positive results.[7]

The use of humor as a deliberate technique by an analyst in individual therapy has been discussed by more recent writers, still with many controversial feelings. Lawrence Kubie warns us that humor has a high potential for destructiveness, that it can be a dangerous weapon, and the mere fact that it amuses and entertains the therapist and gives him a pleasant feeling is not evidence that it is a valuable experience for the patient.[8] His intent, Kubie says, is not to persuade us never to use humor or that it is always destructive, but that this potential should be considered. Humor can be a humanizing influence, ease tension in social situations, and express true warmth and affection, but it is also used to mask hostility and, in the hands of an anxious or junior analyst, can be harmful. Kubie then points out some significant considerations in the use of humor.

Although humor may facilitate the flow of free associations, it may block or arrest the patient's spontaneous stream of thought and may also confuse the patient as to whether the therapist is serious or "only joking." Humor can be used by the analyst as a defense against his own or the patient's anxiety and as a mask for his own hostility. The patient may feel compelled to join in the humor "to be a good sport," thus finding it impossible to express anger or resentment. If the patient uses self-deprecating humor and the therapist joins in, this may deepen the patient's self-deprecating feelings.

Patients also may use humor as a defense against accepting the importance of their own illness. If we laugh, we may reinforce this defense. A gentle, sympathetic humor can be used more appropriately when the treatment process seems to be approaching a successful termination, as one of the signs of improvement, or to mobilize new insight, Kubie concludes.

The critical issue is that it is never justifiable to make fun of or to laugh at the patient or his symptoms. Laughing *with* someone rarely does harm. How to make this distinction may be the most difficult decision to make in the helping process. In the hands of a senior therapist, Kubie says, humor at such times can be a safe and effective tool, but in the hands of a new, inexperienced analyst who may be imitating the senior too early in the game, it may not. Humor, Kubie contends, also impairs the therapist's necessary "incognito" — that is, use of the couch with the doctor sitting behind, with silence, distance, and detachment and no social relationships between patient and analyst, or sharing of analyst's personal life or experiences. The psychotherapeutic relationship is a highly charged one and puts a demand on the psychotherapist for a degree of wisdom and maturity man has not reached, Kubie says. This technical device, placing a distance between patient and doctor, serves to protect the patient from the frailties of the therapist. Humor, he says, "has its place in life. Let's keep it there."

The question is: what *is* its place in life? Is not psychotherapy dealing with the problems of *life* and the patient's living in it! Mindess makes a cogent statement:

The point is that to encourage a humorous outlook in his patients the therapist must keep the dimension alive in himself. If he can perceive the irony in their predicaments and in his own as well, his perception will permeate his interviews and will, when his patients are supple enough to take it, enlarge their comprehension of themselves.

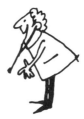

But there — I'm afraid we must confess — 's the rub. A glance at any professional journal, a visit to any professional meeting, make it apparent that psychotherapists take themselves too seriously. We really believe — and the more renowned among us believe it the more — that the theories we propound and the techniques we apply are cogent, valid, and beneficial. Not only do we believe it; we must believe it to be effective. And yet, as long as the belief is maintained, a deep and genuine sense of humor cannot be achieved and therefore promoted. As long as we fail to contemplate the likelihood that our professional activities are useless, that psychotherapy of any sort is absurd in the larger scale of things, we remain bound to the very outlook from which we need to free our patients.[9]

Another analyst, Warren Poland, also reacts negatively to Kubie with the belief that humor can be constructive in psychotherapy and that the incognito technique was devised not to serve as a defense for the analyst, but to frustrate the patient's wish for transference gratification and should be used only to the extent it promotes further psychologic work by the patient. Before using humor, Poland says, the therapist should evaluate the strength of the therapeutic alliance. When humor is integrated, appropriate, and spontaneous, it is indicative of a good therapeutic alliance and informative of the presence of the patient's observing ego. To refute Kubie's statement that therapists never reveal their use of humor, he cites two cases.

In one example, a patient's initial response to the relationship was one of enthusiasm, pleased at everything the analyst had to say. After about two months, this changed to the opposite, with the patient complaining about the analyst, no matter what he did or said:

> At one point in the patient's discourse......he reflected, "I used to hang on your every word." With a laugh [the analyst] spontaneously erupted, "And now I hang on my every word."[10]

The patient laughed and was able to use this interpretation to look at the process.

Another analyst, Gilbert Rose, analyzed humor and pointed out how it may operate beneficially in treatment. First, he says, humor depends on the analyst's personal style. Second, the analyst having a talent for it, the use of humor, like all interventions, depends on the analyst's tact, judgment, and awareness in weighing the effects of the humor at a given moment. Third, the use of humor should always be directed toward a stable therapeutic alliance. Used in this way, Rose says, humor is not an evasion of reality, but an invitation to collaborate to increase awareness. He analyzes specific benefits. Humor may be used to mobilize benign aspects of the superego and support the ego. It may be used to lift repression and render acceptable an interpretation that otherwise cannot be made. It may transmit reality in the right blend of closeness and distance. He gives several examples: The remark to a patient, "If you go on like this, I may have to believe in the unconscious," makes use of the mechanism of negation to convey several interpretations. Light humor may be one way to interpret a sexualized transference resistance. "I'll bet you say that to all your psychiatrists," is an appreciative response to a patient's seductive communication, a recognition that it is just a "line," but the work of treatment will go on. Humor, Rose feels, may play a part in establishing and maintaining a freer interaction between patient and analyst.[11]

This freer interaction and the more open, sharing, reality-oriented approach to the care and treatment of emotionally distressed individuals is reflected in most of the other psychotherapeutic models in recent years. It not only reflects the acceptance of humor as a reality of life and as an integral part of the communication pattern between patient and therapist, and between patient and patient, but also reflects the patient's ability to laugh at himself. "The neurotic who learns to laugh at himself may be on the way to self-management, perhaps to cure."[12] Humanistic and existential psychotherapies reflect this philosophy.

Viktor Frankl has incorporated humor in his method of therapy called *logotherapy*.[13] As a student of Freud, he began his career with a psychoanalytic orientation, but became influenced by the writings of existential philosophers. His philosophy and therapy were tested and strengthened by his experience as a prisoner in a German concentration camp. Frankl found that man can preserve a vestige of spiritual freedom even in such terrible conditions. If there is a meaning to life, there is a meaning to suffering. This will to find meaning is the basic concept of his therapeutic process. His aim is to enable the patient to acquire a new perspective, to rise above the powerful negative driving forces in his life and to a new and true meaning in life. One's sense of self is not seen as fixed but rather one's sense of self is laughed at for its foolish and self-defeating strivings. Humor as the capacity to laugh at oneself is a natural characteristic. This quality of self-detachment in humor is utilized in a procedure Frankl calls *paradoxical intention*. It is based on the concept that what one fears happens, but hyper-intention makes impossible what one wishes. As soon as the patient stops fighting his obsessions or phobias and starts ridiculing or joking about them, the vicious circle is cut and the symptom diminishes and atrophies.

In the therapeutic community approach to psychiatric treatment there is an emphasis on a democratic and human orientation, the use of group psychotherapy, and patient government as well as other social concepts, *i.e.,* patients assuming responsibility for their own behavior, for the welfare of others, and for group living. Within this setting, humor occurs and serves a social as well as psychological function.

The humor used by patients on one such ward in a VA hospital is described by Kaplan and Boyd.[14] They felt that previous studies had ignored those functions of humor aimed at creating a feeling of intimacy and providing a means of winning social approval. Several needs of the patient groups were apparent: to adapt to the staff and others of the wider society; to restrain disruptive tendencies in the group; to alleviate personal anxiety; and to maintain a sense of solidarity.

Several themes in the humor expressed proved to be dominant. One was the "overdependence" allegedly fostered by the "comfortable" life of the VA hospital. The humor here served several functions; it reflected concern over possible maladaptation to the hospital; it assuaged the guilt associated with hospitalization; it reaffirmed the basic value of "wanting to get well"; and it served as an effective negative sanction against those who deviated from this value. The hospital was referred to as "Heroes Hotel," the "Neuropsychiatric Hilton," and the "Federal Womb."

Sex and obscenity was another common theme. Such joking was expected, since this was a male group; the infringement of a social taboo tends to make peer groups more cohesive and has "leveling" influence. It can be used as a "weapon" against the staff, but in such a way that it does not seriously disrupt the system. It also permits the patient group to identify with a normal group (the staff) by projecting on the staff the qualities the patients observe in themselves. One patient claimed he had a sex problem. "I've been screwed by the government for 15 years."

Humor about severe mental disorder was another theme. This humor served to allow dissociation from severe disturbance, and contributed toward cohesiveness and a social control function. However, the patients ridiculed such behavior on other wards, but rarely their own group. Rather, when a disturbance did occur in their group, it was occasion for solicitude and giving of support.

Expressions of hostility through humor were also reported. When directed toward the staff, this kind of humor served as a morale booster among the patients. When expressed toward "civilians" it functioned to decrease the distance and the difference between them. The expression of hostile humor toward other patients helped to forestall deviant behavior and imposed a negative sanction. However, much of the humor directed toward other patients served to enhance the solidarity of the group by functioning as an initiation rite, providing support, and as an expression of comradeship. They called the ward "Thorazine Hilton" and referred to projective tests as "those dirty pictures." When asked by a psychiatrist what he thought about calling doctors by their first names, one patient said, "John, I just don't feel right about calling you John." They controlled behavior of other patients by kidding them about that behavior — "telling tall tales," or being a "firebug." When new patients joined the group, older patients often introduced themselves as the ward psychiatrist or as Sigmund Freud. They played practical jokes on each other. Self-deprecating humor was used by patients either to deny the seriousness of their illness or to "accommodate" the staff. However, it was felt that this self-ridicule permitted the person for the first time to take a detached view of himself and his problem; this recognition is the *sine qua non* of therapeutic process. There seemed to be a relationship between the development of a sense of humor and "getting better."

The authors felt that the beneficial functions as well as the possible dysfunctional consequences of humor should be studied further as a consideration toward the facilitation of therapeutic progress.

Observing humor in group psychotherapy, Vargas saw it used in three ways: (1) to conceal some part of the personality which is considered distressing or undesirable, (2) to facilitate expression, and (3) to disguise yet express a feeling without overt commitment.[15] He further elaborates on these. The patient may use humor to desensitize terms and concepts, to bring about a simple release of tension in the group, to express his judgment of events and conditions in the hospital, to facilitate the discussion of a frightening topic, or to provide the doorway by which he can enter into discussion of a serious problem.

Humor in group psychotherapy also provides a means for controlling deviant behavior.

> In one therapeutic community where group psychotherapy included the total ward, newly admitted patients were simply included and introduced to the group. One day when a new patient was displaying very bizarre behavior, gesturing, posturing, etc., another patient finally leaned out and said to her, "Gladys, in this hospital you can be as crazy as you want, but, you can't act it! So, sit up!" At which point, the group laughed, but the patient sat up!

As there is humor in this setting between patients, so there is humor among staff. As we indicated earlier, in such a stress-provoking setting, humor is common. A study conducted in 1954 analyzed the laughter in psychiatric staff conferences.[16] Group laughter functioned as a mechanism to promote solidarity and provide a safety valve for divisive tensions. The major forms of humor were disparagement and incongruity. The commonest content of the laughter was at physicians and patients. There was a low percentage of laughter at sexual themes, but a heartiness of laughter at death. The social function of the laughter seemed to vary with the situation, *e.g.,* a need for group tension release, uncertainty over a controversial issue, expression of a need for emotional support or to secure status, or a response to a violation of mores or of objective reality. The disparagement of patients by the staff, which relieved their tensions and served the well-being of the group, placed a barrier between the patient and the personnel. Those listening to the case tended to lose sight of the disease process in the patient. This withdrawal from the patient's problems was deemed by the observers as an inappropriate response in view of therapeutic responsibilities.

Yet the relief from a difficult situation is as necessary for the staff as for the patient. In the milieu of a psychiatric hospital, Coser says, where the therapeutic process requires interactive competency, a staff member's every-day behavior has to be carefully controlled by himself and others.[17] The self-consciousness and tension that arise under these conditions may seek release through humor.

In her study of the social functions of humor among the staff of a mental hospital during staff meetings, Coser found that humor among colleagues served to reduce the social distance, to relax the rigidity of the social structure without upsetting it. It served as a means of mutual reassurance, of asking for and giving support, of teaching and learning, of affirmation of common values in an area fraught with uncertainties.

Within the hierarchy of an organization like this mental hospital, she found the status structure was supported by downward humor. That is, those high in the hierarchy felt free to make the most witticisms, while those lowest on the authority structure made the fewest. Most of the witticisms were directed at some target: a patient, relatives, another staff member, or self. The least use of humor by those low on the staff did not mean they had less hostility and less need, but rather pointed out that role relationships within a situation control the behavior. The junior staff members were supposed to learn, to receive knowledge and to accept the intellectual superiority of the senior members. Too much humorous behavior would be interpreted as questioning the student-teacher relationship. The most frequent targets of the senior staff were the junior members, while the junior members directed their humor against patients, relatives, or themselves. Never was the humor within the meeting directed at an authority higher than the initiators.

Self-deprecating humor by a junior member, using himself as a target, pays respect to the system, but also decreases the social distance, since he permits authority an expression of its own aggression through laughter. The laughter of the authority figure grants the junior member's plea for belongingness and strengthens the cohesion of the group.

Humor and laughter in the group may also dramatize a violation of a norm and at the same time reaffirm that norm. The humorist assumes the role of disguised moralist. The individual with a high staff position most often uses this role as a teaching device. The junior uses humor as a means of self-protection, a plea for sympathy. The laughter and humorous responses by the authority figure and the group combine criticism with support. This kind of humor informs the junior that it is not serious, they they can all laugh about it together, yet at the same time points out the violation or blunder.

The junior member is in a paradoxical position. He has

to assume the role of a student with his seniors, but to be a successful student, he must assume a professional, nonstudent role with his patients. The paradox may seek its solution in self-aggressive humor and humor about patients which is not aggression against patients, but gets him the support and reassurance he needs, because it is an area around which consensus is easy. Coser says:

> The need for support is great indeed for those who have to deal with illness, especially in an area in which results are slow to be forthcoming and in which the therapist must constantly scrutinize and evaluate the techniques at his disposal.[18]

Humor is used as a device for lending support and for asking for support.

> The give and take of support through humor helps the participants to live up to role expectations and to overcome the contradictions and ambiguities inherent in the complex social structure, and therapy to contribute to its maintenance.[19]

The implications, then, for the education of the health professional through the use of humor are great. To reiterate O'Connell's statement: to achieve the necessary professional maturity, potential psychiatrists may need education toward increased empathy and humor. There is a need, he said, for "empathetic tutoring by exemplary figures to further develop empathy and humor.[20]

The relevance to education for all health professionals in all areas can be extrapolated from this base. In the next chapter we will attempt to describe this concept of humor in relation to the educational process of the health professional.

REFERENCES

1. O'Connell WE, Rothhous P, Hansen PG, Moyer R: Jest appreciation and interaction in leaderless groups. *International Journal of Group Psychotherapy* 19:454-462, 1969.
2. *Ibid*, p 454.
3. O'Connell WE, Covert C: Death attitudes and humor appreciation among medical students. *Existential Psychiatry*, p 433-442, Winter 1967, p 436.
4. Zwerling I: The favorite joke in diagnostic and therapeutic interviewing. *Psychoanalytic Quarterly* 24:104-114, 1955.

5. Brody MW: The meaning of laughter. *Psychoanalytic Quarterly* 19:193-201, 1950.
6. Nussbaum K, Michaux W: Response to humor in depression: a predictor and evaluator of patient change? *Psychiatric Quarterly* 37:527-539, 1963.
7. Robinson VM: Humor in nursing. *In* Carlson C (ed): pp 143-44.
8. Kubie LS: The destructive potential of humor in psychotherapy. *American Journal of Psychiatry* 127:861-866, 1971.
9. Mindess H: *Laughter and Liberation,* p 220.
10. Poland WS: The place of humor in psychotherapy. *American Journal of Psychiatry* 128:127-129, 1971.
11. Rose GJ: King Lear and the use of humor in treatment. *Journal of the American Psychoanalytic Association* 12:927-940, 1969.
12. Allport GW: *The Individual and His Religion.* New York, The Macmillan Co, 1950, p 92.
13. Frankl V: *Man's Search for Meaning.* New York, Washington Square Press, 1963.
14. Kaplan H, Boyd IH: The social functions of humor on an open psychiatric ward. *Psychiatric Quarterly* 39:502-15, 1965.
15. Vargas MJ: Uses of humor in group psychotherapy. *Group Psychotherapy* 14:198-202, 1961.
16. Goodrich AT, Jules H, Goodrich DW: Laughter in psychiatric conferences: a sociopsychiatric analysis. *Am J Orthopsychiatry* 24:175-184, 1954.
17. Coser RL: Laughter among colleagues. *Psychiatry* 23:81-95, February, 1960.
18. *Ibid,* p 91.
19. *Ibid,* p 95.
20. O'Connell, *Death Attitudes,* p 441.

BIBLIOGRAPHY

Mosak HH, Dreikurs R: Adlerian psychotherapy. *In* Corsini R (ed): *Current Psychotherapies.* Itasca, Illinois, FE Peacock Publishers, 1973, p 53.

O'Connell WE: Humor and death. *Psychological Reports* 22:391-402, 1968.

O'Connell WE: Resignation, humor and wit. *Psycho Analytic Review* 51:49-56, 1964.

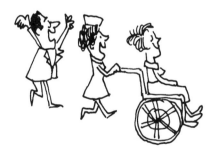

humor in
ed+u×ca=tion

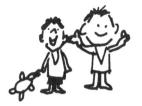

The Perception of the Comic is a tie of sympathy with other men, a pledge of sanity. We must learn by laughter as well as by tears and terror.

RALPH WALDO EMERSON

Another of the benefits of humor which has been identified by many is that of facilitating or enhancing learning. "What is learned with laughter is learned well."[1] Marshall McLuhan says:

> Learning, the educational process, has long been associated only with the glum. We speak of the 'serious' student. Our time presents a unique opportunity for learning by means of humor — a perceptive or incisive joke can be more meaningful than platitudes lying between two covers.[2]

Carl Rogers states that a sense of humor is one of the essential qualities of that facilitator of learning, the teacher.[3]

Despite the recognition of its importance, however, there has been little attempt by educators to make conscious, deliberate use of humor in the educational setting.

The use of humor in the classroom by the teacher not only enhances learning and fosters the student-teacher relationship, but can provide the vehicle for developing the student's ability to relate in this warm and human way to others. The modeling of the use of humor by the instructor is also a first step in teaching the student in the helping professions how to utilize humor as a communication tool in intervening with patients in times of stress.

The socialization of the student into the health profession begins the day he enters his first classroom. As we have discussed previously, he learns very quickly that humor is one way to cope with the "reality shocks" he encounters. The educational system has a responsibility to assist in this socialization process and it must assume responsibility for helping the student learn to use this humor in an acceptable and constructive way.

There are four interrelated aspects, then, to be considered in this area of education and humor:

1. Enhancing the learning process itself through humor.
2. Facilitating the process of socialization into the health profession through humor
3. Teaching the concept of humor as a communication tool.
4. Modeling the use of humor as a vehicle for facilitating the other three.

There are no known empirical studies which prove conclusively that humor enhances learning. According to Keith-Spiegel, neither is there any theoretical paper which fits humor into an established learning model, although there are three unpublished doctoral dissertations (Byrne, 1957; Fisher, 1964; Keith-Spiegel, 1968) which have applied the Hullian model to humor appreciation expectancies.

That humor must be a quality of any learning theory and certainly a necessary ingredient in learning *about* learning theories is the basis for Guy R. Lefrancois' book, *Psychological Theories and Human Learning: Kongor's Report.* The book is written as a report by an extraterrestrial being named Kongor M-III 216,784,912,lVKX4 from the planet Koros. (Lefrancois "only collects the royalties.") The chapter describing

Hull's behavoristic system is typical of the humorous manner in which the book is written. (A writing style most authors, including this one, wish they had!)

The system is replete with symbols and mathematical terms and values. While the mathematical terms are not essential to this discussion, the symbols simplify the presentation of the theory — although they do impose some strain on memory. On several occasions, Léfrancois had to take special precautions to prevent "symbol shock" from occurring in undergraduate classes being exposed to Hull's theory for the first time. These precautions consist largely of indelicate stories (told in a delicate manner so as not to offend) interspersed with good Hullian terminology. Symptoms of symbol shock include lower respiration rate, some lowering of body temperature, a change in EEG pattern from Beta to Alpha waves, and closed eyelids. On occasion, some sufferers make strange noises through their mouths. These students are probably in more extreme states of shock.[4]

Kongor himself makes no apologies for the "indelicate" stories or words used but says in the Earth version one particular WORD is used as a pedagogical device because Hull's theoretical position may prove somewhat difficult for the average Earth reader. He goes on to say:

I find it highly amusing that what was included in the Koron version as a piece of humor (on Koros the absurd is comic) should become an essential instructional device on Earth. Of course, we have no "bulls" on Koros; the WORD is therefore slightly different in the Koron version.[5]

Although Lefrancois used humor very effectively in teaching learning theory, he did not relate the concept of humor per se to the framework of any learning theory.

It would seem, then, that rather than a relationship to one particular theory of learning, there is more of the recognition that humor and laughter contribute to all those necessary principles of learning, regardless of theory: enjoyment; interest; motivation; creativity; a relaxed, open, warm atmosphere; a positive student-teacher relationship; and reduced tension and anxiety.

Each of us subjectively can recall or relate some learning which "we will never forget" because it was presented in a humorous manner. The classic definition of menstruation as "the weeping of a disappointed uterus" not only produces a laugh, but conveys the physiology of the menstrual cycle in one short sentence to which the student can always relate!

Actually, if one were to relate humor to a particular learning theory, the humanistic approach to education would probably be the most appropriate. The humanistic perspective is looking toward man's capacity, what he can become rather than the normal, average, or adjusted individual. It is seeking to look at the here and now and the conscious self as opposed to the past orientation and the unconscious of the Freudians, and to looking at what is going on inside the behavior rather than the observable behavior alone as the behaviorists do. Behavior from the humanistic stance is a result of our perceptions. What we perceive about ourselves constitutes our self-concept and affects how we behave. Similarly how we perceive others colors our interactions with them. Building a positive self-image, identifying that self-actualized man and how one produced him, exploring the meanings that lead to behavior, and finding meaning in one's life are the goals of the humanistic movement.

The implications for education are apparent, producing a fully functioning, self-actualized individual and mobilizing the potentials of every student. The teacher then becomes a facilitator of learning, not a director or information giver. He is a warm, caring person who is open, and provides the atmosphere in which the student can be involved in his own becoming and in developing a positive self-concept. The climate of the school from administrators to student is one of open communication, a respect for each other. Individualized instruction, self-pacing, self-discovery, self-management, learning from mistakes, fostering creativity, flexibility, and encouraging the development of personal meaning in learning are all techniques of the humanistic approach to education.

Abraham Maslow, who pioneered the humanistic movement has defined that self-actualized man as having a philosophical, unhostile sense of humor, the ability not only to poke fun at himself, but having a sense of humor which reminds others of their "humanness." He defines humor and laughter as "education in a palatable form."[6]

Being real and genuine is one of the qualities or attitudes of a teacher who facilitates learning, and having a sense of humor is an aspect of being genuine, says Carl Rogers. He quotes a student's reaction: "Your sense of humor in the class was cheering; we all felt relaxed because you showed us your human self, not a mechanical image."[7]

Kenneth Eble in his book, *The Perfect Education*, says laughter creates the very air in which learning thrives. He feels laughter must begin in the home and continue throughout education. Laughter frees up and opens pathways to creativity and discovery. He beseeches parents to shake off the habit of excessive worry and pushing.

> More positively, they must laugh greatly. For children, solemnity is like a whole pane of glass in an abandoned building. Solemnity invites shattering....
>
> But why laughter? Because laughter is giving and recognizing. It forces a physical giving that releases for a moment the very self. And if we did not recognize some rugged corner of ourselves, some flawed reality, we would not laugh. Such giving is necessary to prepare the self to learn.... Parents can hardly do better than respond to

their children's sense of absurdity, to let physical ticklings grow into wit, to let wit grow into a sense of the world as it is and as it should be.[8]

He advises parents to consider laughter even before love because laughter keeps love from smothering, and if we laugh, we are bound to love. He says "...laughter makes parenthood bearable...." If laughter is not linked with learning at home, the connection is not likely to be made in school.

Surely the thing that drives hundreds of bright, laughing college students out of the colleges of education is the solemnity of their utterances as well as their behavior.[9]

Education [should] keep us alive and hopeful...and lead us to laugh in the face of heaven or hell. For serious as our strivings are, they should never be so serious that we cannot lean back and laugh at the absurdity of our being and doing. Education should teach us to play the wise fool rather than turn us into the solemn ass.[10]

The concepts inherent in the humanistic approach to education are ones that have been closely related to the concept of humor. The perception of ourselves and how others perceive us, the loving, caring, warm atmosphere, and the concepts of creativity and change are evidenced in both.

The use of humor is a mechanism which does not destroy one's self-image, but provides a way to criticize, show mistakes, express values yet save face for the individual and imply a loving relationship in doing so. *It's all right. You made a mistake, just something to laugh about, to learn from. No harm done. You are not a terrible person, just human.* Coser, in the study of humor between colleagues (discussed in the previous chapter), describes this use of humor as a teaching device which not only helps to resolve the paradoxical role of the student, who, to be a good student must also be a professional, but also serves as an informal process of socialization into the profession.

The teacher relating humorous experiences of his own

which often show "boo-boos" and mistakes he has made helps the student, who usually has unrealistic expectations of his own performance, to relax and accept the learning process.

The students' imitations and mimickings of instructors and hospital staff (a common practice in health professions), not only in private but at school parties where the subjects of the humor are present, demonstrate the relationship in reverse, that is, the students are able to express their own hostility, to criticize and relieve their anxiety and tension, yet show affection and warmth. Many of the "scenes" in the acting reveal the areas around which the most anxiety for the student has taken place. A clue for the educator to heed in future teaching! These humorous plays and skits also are part of the socialization process. "We're one of you now. We can laugh about it with you!" The student who can initiate humor comfortably with faculty gives evidence of an interpersonal skill that will be reflected in his ability to relate to other people.

The concepts of creativity and change are closely related to each other as well as to humor and learning. Creativity implies the ability to change and produce change. To be a change agent implies the ability to be creative.

> We are...faced with an entirely new situation in education where the goal of education, if we are to survive, is the facilitation of change and learning. The only man who is educated is the man who has learned how to learn...how to adapt to change...realized that no knowledge is secure, that only the process of seeking knowledge gives a basis for security.[11]

The humorous release, says Mindess, is:

> ...change of venue...the sober citizen having gotten the point of a jest, merely exchanges his ordinary outlook for a broader, subtler, or more novel one. Breaking loose from one set, we settle for another...the delight is in the process, in the experience of change.[12]

To cultivate our sense of humor, Mindess goes on to say, requires that we learn to thrive on change.

The aspect of creativity in both learning and humor is obvious. The very act of producing humor or comedy is creativity in itself. Koestler and Fry both speak of humor as an act of creation which requires the ability to abstract and conceptualize. Enjoyment of humor, to get the point of a joke, requires the same ability. The procedure of humor is the procedure for creativity,

> ...for in its construction as well as its content, the ludicrous continually provides us with new compositions formed out of old raw materials...as a body of activity our indulgence in humor facilitates our creative possibilities, for it lubricates the unconventional, imaginative problem-solving functions of our being.[13]

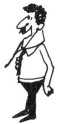

It "paves the way for originality on a wider scale" and "has the power to unlock all our other creative potentials," Mindess concludes.

We have suggested that the educational process begins the socialization of the student, through the use of humor, into the "reality shocks" he faces. In our teaching in those areas which create the social conflicts both student and patient face, a bit of humor facilitates an understanding and may even lead to a discussion of these conflicts.

For example, a comment used by an instructor in a lecture to beginning nursing students, "On Monday we will have a discussion of vomiting, including a practical demonstration of the technique," not only produces a laugh, but in effect says, "I know vomiting isn't a pleasant subject or one which you have been in the habit of dealing with, so let's laugh a little about it." There could follow, then, a discussion of the student's reaction, the patient's reaction, and the responsibilities of a professional in managing this unpleasant situation.

Similarly, in a class on the procedure of giving of an enema, one instructor began her discussion of the psychosocial implications with, "How would you approach a patient to whom you are giving an enema? Would you say, 'Ha! Ha! Look what I've got for you!'?" The students' laughter is acknowledgment of their anxiety in facing the embarrassment and conflict of this situation. Acceptance of humor as one way of coping can be discussed as well as recognizing that the patient may also joke in the situation, and that the student can feel comfortable in responding. Serious discussion of all the implications involved in this procedure as well as others can ensue.

One of the contentions of many educators is that education is a "serious" business, and that scientific and medical subjects, particularly, do not lend themselves to humor. However, this has been refuted by many authors. Even "dull," somber, scientific subjects can be lightened by humor. It is a fallacy that there are "proper" subjects for jokes, while others are too sacred to talk about. It is the time and place which are the decisive factors, not the subject.

A recent textbook on the use of computers in data processing in education in discussing the use of base 10 in mathematics says:

> There is nothing particularly sacred about a base of 10.
> Probably the only reason it was originally developed and is
> now in widespread use is that man happens to have 10

fingers. Other systems have been created. For example, the Babylonians had a base of 60 (of course, they also did their writing on mud pies); the Mayas of Yucatan used a base of 20 (warm climate and groups of barefooted mathematicians?); and a base of five is still used by natives in New Hebrides (one hand is wrapped around a spear and is thus not available for counting?).[14]

In the medical field, not all situations or human diseases lend themselves to humor, but, even there a relatively somber, scientific discussion as to why the sphincter ani must be preserved when performing surgery in that area was described by Bornemeier in an amusing style:

They say man has succeeded where the animal fails because of the clever use of his hands, yet when compared to the hands, the sphincter ani is far superior. If you place into your cupped hands a mixture of fluid, solid and gas and then through an opening at the bottom, try to let only the gas escape, you will fail. Yet the sphincter ani can do it. The sphincter apparently can differentiate between solid, fluid and gas. It apparently can tell whether its owner is alone or with someone, whether standing up or sitting down, whether its owner has his pants on or off. No other muscle in the body is such a protector of the dignity of man, yet so ready to come to his relief. A muscle like this is worth protecting.[15]

Robert Baker, who believes that science and humor are not mutually contradictory, has put together a collection of scientific humor in a book entitled, *A Stress Analysis of a Strapless Evening Gown and Other Essays for a Scientific Age.* The essays include such intriguing titles as "The Lab Coat as Status Symbol" by F.E. Warburton; "Parkinson's Laws in Medical Research" by C. Northcote Parkinson; "Saga of a New Hormone" by Norman Applezweig; and "Body Ritual Among the Nacirema" by Horace Miner. Baker says

...both scientists and satirists [are] dedicated to the proposition that neither science nor man can hope to survive the rigors of our age without a sense of humor.[16]

Another collection of humorous essays by Baker is called *Psychology in the Wry*.[17] It was assembled, he says, because too many professional psychologists and their students have not only forgotten how to laugh, but also believe it is unscientific to do so! The contributors represent many branches of psychology, and have created this new branch, a science of satire, in defense of psychology's mental health! One article entitled, "Sidesteps Toward a Nonspecial Theory" by Edgar F. Borgatta, presents some theories Freud overlooked: deumbilification, mammary envy, digital gratification, and the no-person group.

When teaching in a scientific, somber, or delicate area such as health or disease, one must always balance between achievement of a goal and a need for tact in the use of the humor to avoid misunderstandings and offending sensibilities. Yet, as Reese sums up the case for humor in medicine:

> I would never suggest that the physician writer not take his medicine seriously. I do hope, however, he will occasionally laugh at himself, amuse his readers when it helps to get and hold their attention, warm up his facts before he serves them, and use humor whenever it adds a touch of humanity.[18]

In this chapter, we have expressed a belief that humor does have a valuable place in education. How the educator can learn to model it and teach the use of humor as a tool in communication will be discussed in *Section III, Cultivating the Use of Humor.*

REFERENCES

1. Grotjahn M: *Beyond Laughter,* p ix.
2. McLuhan M: *The Medium is the Massage.* New York, Bantam Books, 1967, p 10.
3. Rogers C: *Freedom to Learn.* Columbus, Ohio, Charles E. Merrill, 1969, p 108.
4. Lefrancois GR: *Psychological Theories and Human Learning: Kongor's Report.* Monterey Calif., Brooks/Cole Publishing Co, 1972, p 124.
5. *Ibid,* p 122-23.
6. Maslow AH: *Motivation and Personality,* 2nd ed. New York, Harper and Row, 1970, pp 169-170.
7. Rogers, *Freedom to Learn,* p 108.

8. Eble KE: *A Perfect Education.* New York, The Macmillan Co, 1966, p 4.
9. *Ibid,* p 15.
10. *Ibid,* p 214.
11. Rogers, *Freedom to Learn,* p 104.
12. Mindess, *Laughter and Liberation,* p 142.
13. *Ibid,* p 153-54.
14. Sanders OH: *Computers in Society.* New York, McGraw-Hill, 1973, p 147.
15. Bornemeier WC: Sphincter protecting hemorroidectomy. *Am J Proctocology* 11:48-52, 1960.
16. Baker RA: *A Stress Analysis of a Strapless Evening Gown and Other Essays for a Scientific Age.* Englewood Cliffs, New Jersey, Prentice-Hall, 1967, p ix.
17. Baker RA: *Psychology in the Wry.* Princeton, New Jersey, D. Van Nostrand Co, Inc. 1963.
18. Reese RL: Does humor have a place in scientific writing? *Am Med Writer's Assoc Bull* 17:11-13, 1967.

BIBLIOGRAPHY

Perceiving Behaving Becoming: A New Focus for Education. Washington, D.C., National Education Association, Association for Supervision and Curriculum Development, Yearbook, 1962.

Mikes G: *Laughing Matter.* New York, The Library Press, 1971.

Olendzki M: *Cautionary Tales.* Wakefield, Mass, Contemporary Publishing Co, 1973.

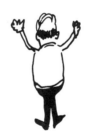

humor related to Culture and illness

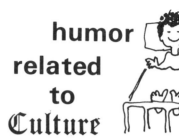

One of the variables always to be considered in planning health care is the cultural background of the patient and family. Each culture has practices and beliefs which influence the reaction to illness and to health care. Health personnel must be as sensitive to the cultural needs of people as they are to the physical, psychological, and social needs. "Today, more than ever before, there is a need to understand people from different cultures and to use this knowledge in the helping process."[1]

> Cultural differences are often the basis for poor communication, interpersonal tensions, and hesitation in working effectively with others. Cultural similarities make us appreciate humanness, common human bonds, and behavior features which point to human universality.[2]

The humor within cultures, and the similarities and differences, then, must also be a factor to be considered in the planned use of humor in interactions with patients and their families. Is there a difference in the kind of humor which emanates from a particular culture or ethnic group? Does culture or ethnicity make a difference in the kind of humor which is appreciated? Are there similarities or are there universal topics for humor? Is there a relationship between a specific culture and its use of humor in times of stress like illness? If so, what is it?

Would the culture of the patient make a difference in the health professional's use of humor if the professional were a nonmember of the culture?

Definitive answers to these questions, as with most others in this area of humor, are not available. There are the same varied opinions and generalizations. Specific studies regarding humor and cultural or ethnic groups are rare and comprehensive studies regarding cultural groups and their use of humor in relation to health and illness, are apparently nonexistent.

We know little that is fundamental about national and ethnic differences in human behavior. Yet we know that smiling and laughter transcend cultures and that humor is a molding force in all societies. The popular humor of a people often expresses their concerns, conflicts and aspirations. We can hypothesize that there will be differences, but that there will also be similarities since laughter is a universal human behavior.

This dichotomy of humor is illustrated by the Greenland Eskimos who resolve their quarrels by duels of laughter. Each recites humorous insults and obscene jokes ridiculing his opponent. The one who gets the most laughs from the audience wins. The other, humiliated, often goes into exile.

Some types of humor, however, seem to transcend cultures. Charlie Chaplin, during a visit to a primitive tribe in East Africa, was expected to respond in kind after their dance performance for him. He chose to dance for them his pantomine of a bullfight. The natives roared with laughter. He then went one step farther, and performed a bedroom farce of a woman caught by her husband in bed with her lover. This act also was understood and resulted in hilarity.

Nearly every society has developed some form of institutionalized humor as a method of social release and regulation. Radcliffe-Brown in 1940 first described the "joking relationship" from his study of primitive tribes in

Africa. This social relationship has been found to be widespread in all societies. He defined the term as "a relation between two persons in which one is by custom permitted, and in some instances required, to tease or make fun of the other, who in turn is required to take no offense."³ There are two varieties. In the symmetrical, both participants can tease and make fun of each other. In the asymmetrical, one teases the other who either can accept it good-humoredly without retaliating or only teases back a little. In some instances, the joking and teasing are only verbal; in others there is horse-play, and still others include elements of obscenity. The joking relationship is a peculiar combination of friendliness and antagonism. It is one of "permitted disrespect." This is important, Levine says, because the "maintenance of a social order depends upon the appropriate kind and degree of respect being shown towards certain persons, things and ideas or symbols."⁴

This teasing and joking relationship performs a vital function in defining and maintaining kinship relationships. It also provides the culture with external controls for the sexual and aggressive urges that would violate the rules of that culture if expressed directly. In many of our American Indian tribes the ritual clown is a highly respected individual who, in his antics as part of the ceremonies of the tribe, is permitted to violate every social taboo. Such a relationship provides a vicarious release for the audience.

Although no studies have shown clear differences in the humor of various nationalities and ethnic groups, we nevertheless identify various types of jokes by their ethnic character. We speak of Irish jokes, Jewish jokes, Scottish jokes, German jokes, English jokes, etc. These jokes may reveal the personality or character traits, the stereotypes or the conflicts of that particular group. These may be reflected in the style of humor or the content. One study found German humor full of sympathetic feeling, English humor attempting to fight off seriousness, American humor primitive and full of exaggerations which seem silly to the Germans, and French wit as cruel and hostile. Later investigators found no real differences.

Mikes feels that people all over the world laugh at the same things, but there are some jokes which reflect the national character. A crook or cheat is always portrayed as fair in an English joke, whereas he is clever in a Jewish joke. The victim is seen as stupid in the German version of the joke. Understatement is the style of the British; overstatement, exaggeration, and leg-pulling characterize the style of the American. The love of self-mockery and self-criticism is shared by both English and Jews.

The Jews needed jokes, Mikes contends. It was the only way they could survive through thousands of years of persecution, the only way to save their self-respect and to laugh at their tormentors. There are many jokes about anti-Semitism and superior Jewish cleverness. This is a preventative mechanism that wards off anticipated attack, has pride as well as humility, and pleads for love. It creates for the Jews a bond and a solidarity. Tell a Jewish joke to an anti-Semite, Mikes contends, and if he laughs he will be less anti-Semitic. A reflection of the change in their social situation, Jewish humor, he says, has been lost in transit to Israel. Jews in Israel are no longer oppressed! Humor still survives, but the difference is seen in this joke:

An Israeli couple is touring Europe with their 11-year-old child. He asks in Italy, Germany, Holland, Sweden,

"Are these people Jews?" He is told each time, "No, they are Christians." The boy, with sympathy, finally says, "Poor Christians. It must be awful for them to be scattered like that all over the world."[5]

Humor has served similar functions for other minority cultures. Many comedians and analysts of comedy claim that humor has done more to change the status of minority groups and reduce racial prejudice than any other factor. The television program, *Laugh-In*, did much to return ethnic humor to good standing. Evidence of the change may be the popularity of current TV shows like *Good Times, Sanford and Son, All in the Family, The Jeffersons,* and *Chico and the Man.* Black comedians like Dick Gregory and Ossie Davis feel wit and humor are better weapons and a greater force than anger in easing racial tension.

Investigation of humor in relation to the issue of racial prejudice in minority cultures has been the focus of several studies and writings over the years. Myrdal, in the context of race relations, described a number of social functions provided by intergroup humor: as an escape route, as compensation to the sufferer, as absolution provided in the form of an understanding laugh, and as indirect approval for that which cannot be explicitly acknowledged.[6]

In the history of racial conflict humor has played a definite role.[7] It lends itself well to use as a conflict device because of its boundless limits in subject matter and because its nature is such that it often contains more or less well-concealed malice. Burma discusses particularly Negro-White humor which makes one or the other the butt of the humor. The notion of Negroes lampooning Whites may come as a surprise. Yet for many decades Negroes were usually in a position in which their conflict and defense techniques had to be covert. This favored the growth of a more subtle type of humor as a weapon of both offense and defense.

Prejudice, both racial and cultural, provides a fertile field for the folklorist. Folktales created by minority groups toward whom prejudice is shown function through sarcasm, humor, or parody to preserve the ego identity of the minority group. This type of humor conserves mental health through sublimation, allowing release of the suppressed anger via protest humor.

These tales utilize several techniques. One may state that personal salvation is to be found only within the minority group and that anyone who adopts the customs of the majority group is lost. Another tale may involve trickster motifs by which a member of the group successfully counters an insult by the majority group. Another may parody an alleged stereotype or follow a majority group logic to an unexpected conclusion. A fifth may denigrate the majority group.

In summary, humor functions in intergroup conflict as a mechanism for expressing aggression toward an out-group through the use of sarcasm and ridicule, enhancing the morale of the in-group and undermining the morale of those against whom the humor is directed. In addition, humor may serve as a means of accommodation, as the Negro slave appeased his white master through self-ridicule and self-debasement.

A STUDY OF THREE CULTURES

If comprehensive studies and analyses of humor in specific cultures are rare, the use of humor in times of illness in specific cultures is even more rare. To provide some beginning base for consideration of the variable of cultures in using humor as a tool in communication, a concentration on a small number of cultures was thought to be more fruitful. The problem was approached by looking first for specific studies of humor in that culture, and then reviewing the literature on health and illness in that culture in an attempt to find any references to the use of humor, or any correlations between the two. As a third step, a small study was conducted to attempt to collect some original data.

Since national humor (Irish, Scottish, French, English, German, and the like) has been more or less accepted and incorporated into the Anglo-Saxon melting pot of our western culture, it was felt that reviewing specific minority cultures within our American society would be more meaningful. Consequently, the three cultures: Black-American, Spanish-American, and Southwest Indian were chosen. Each would have, as a similar component, the use of humor as a minority group.

The *Southwest Indian* was chosen since there are differences recognized by anthropologists and linguists between various Indian groups. In the Southwest Indian group, the literature relates more specifically to the Navajo.

Spanish-American and *Black-American* are compromise terms and are used in a broad sense to define those two groups. There are many distinctions made and many individual preferences expressed.

Leininger makes a distinction between Spanish-Americans who are descendents of the Spanish colonists, the Mexican-Americans who migrated from Mexico, and the Mexicans. Each have their own heritage and differences, yet there are similarities in belief and all are Spanish-speaking. Nava separates the Mexican-American from other Spanish-surnamed, stating that they represent several races and different cultures. Most

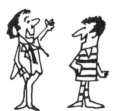

are mestizos, part Spanish and part Indian, but some are pure Indian and some pure Spanish. The younger generation today prefer to be called *Chicano,* reflecting the more aggressive stance, rejecting assimilation into the Anglo culture and demanding respect for their bicultural identity. Individuals differ widely in their preferences. Some prefer *Spanish-American,* others, *Mexican-American* or *Hispano, Latino* or *Chicano.* Some reject the term *Chicano* because of its militant connotation. Others prefer either the *Spanish* or *Mexican* term, reflecting whether they feel their heritage is Spanish or Mexican.

Similarly, in the Black-American group, there are variations. Some groups prefer *Afro-American* rather than *Black,* reflecting their African heritage. *Negro* is still used in many studies as an anthropological term, even though *Black* has become a widely preferred term, adopted by the new generation in their militant movement to gain equality and respect. "Black is beautiful." Here again, there are individual preferences. One very indignant young lady said to me: "I am Negro! See that skin? It's not black! And, I don't dress, think, or act like the 'Blacks.'" However, terms like *colored* are universally resented.

Because of the association of most of these terms with *minority,* which can perpetuate the feelings of inferiority and discrimination, the Western Council on Higher Education for Nursing is suggesting that the term *Ethnic groups of color* be used to begin to create a change in attitude. In the exploratory study conducted by this author, the terms *Black-American, Spanish-American,* and *Indian-American* were established after preliminary discussions with various groups and individuals. In every pre- and post-interview, reactions to these terms were solicited. Often a spontaneous reaction occurred prior to the discussion. One individual also reacted to the term *Anglo* as discriminatory.

The exploratory study was designed to collect humorous incidents in health settings when the patient was from one of these three cultures. The purpose was to provide some beginning data to answer the question of whether the culture of the patient makes a difference in the use of humor by the patient or health professional.

Three health agencies agreed to participate in the study: a large general hospital in the inner city area, a public health agency in a predominantly black residential district, and a neighborhood health center in a predominantly Spanish-American community. Despite the enthusiasm of the 60 health professionals who agreed to collect data, only 15 actual incidents were reported. The study suffered from the same problems of investigation described in the first chapter. Information gathered in pre- and post-interviews provided many more recollections of incidents which had occurred in the past, as well as personal opinions and thoughts regarding the differences and similarities.

Southwest Indian

Of the three groups, the Indian culture is the only one in which an anthropological study of humor has been conducted. Extensive studies of the Navajo Indian culture were done in the 1940s.

> A popular fallacy has long existed that the American Indian is a stolid, unemotional individual incapable of expression or appreciation of humor or wit. Nothing is farther from the truth. Examples taken from the Navaho show that in his own social sphere the Indian can and does scintillate in conversation and in action in a manner comparable to that of peoples of European cultures. His humor runs the gamut of puns, practical jokes, and obscenities. In addition, he is an excellent mimic and pantomimist with a superb sense of timing and climax.[8]

Others describe the Navajo's keen sense of humor as having a whimsical quality that is seldom cruel. Wit and repartee are highly valued in conversation. Between relatives, a patterned type of teasing occurs. All types of humor are indulged in and reacted to by all classes and ages of persons. There is less difference due to age, sex, and social position than in white society. A respected older man often acts the buffoon. However, the Navajo does not like to be laughed at, and he wants to be well regarded by his white friends particularly.

The importance of laughter as a social communication device can be illustrated by the practice of providing a festive meal for the family prepared by the person who elicits a baby's first laugh. It is marked as a milestone and occasion in the baby's life.

The clown is a very important institution in the Navajo culture and is a vital part of the religious rituals. Religion and illness are very closely related and medicine or treatment is administered with much ceremony by the clowns who are impersonating the gods. The ritualistic process ejects the evil and the good is absorbed by the patient. A person subjected to a ceremony thus possesses a great many powers to keep him safe. Sandpainting is one such ceremony in which the sand absorbs the evil and the patient absorbs the good of the supernaturals represented by the sand.

The study conducted by Kluckhohn and Leighton was an analysis of the Indian Service program in the 1930s. The shortcomings of the program were a result of the failure to understand the cultural patterns of the Navajo. The health program particularly was adversely affected by not taking into consideration the beliefs around illness and disease.

Among the beliefs is the idea that the individual is a unit; therefore, parts of the body should not be treated separately. The Navajo "Singers" or medicine men, who cured with rituals, treated patients accordingly whereas white doctors were apt to treat specific illnesses. That nature is more powerful than man is a theme which pervades the whole culture, and the supernatural fears and beliefs extend to illness and disease. There is a belief that by witchcraft evil men and women can produce the illness or death of those whom they hate. Since there is no belief in immortality, death and everything connected with it are abhorred by the Navajo. There is a fear of ghosts, the dead who may return to plague the living. Therefore a disease or injury is not caused by some physiological process, but rather by a violation of one of the taboos or beliefs, by a ghost or by witchcraft. The treatment then is to appease the supernaturals. The aim of the curing ceremonials is to restore the patient to a normal condition in his supernatural relationships. The Navajo values highly health and strength, and fears disease and injury. However, he rarely shares his beliefs with the white man because they are sacred and not to be readily shared with just anyone.

It is a great disappointment to the Indian people that the granite-faced grunting redskin stereotype still has been perpetuated, says Vine Deloria, a Sioux.[9] Indians have found a humorous side to nearly every problem, he says, and use teasing as a method for controlling social situations. Today, humor occupies a prominent place in national Indian affairs. Tribes are brought together by sharing humor of the past. "Columbus" jokes gain great sympathy as well as jokes about the Bureau of Indian Affairs and General Custer. Tribes enjoy teasing each other. They agree that humor is the cement that holds the Indian movement together.

Vine Deloria speaks for the New Indian, who is no longer fighting for physical survival; he is fighting for ideological survival. The new generation of university-educated Indians has given voice to a human morality and tribal philosophy of life that weds the ancient with the modern. These young educated Indians are going back to be tribal leaders, to teach, to practice medicine and nursing, and to build educational facilities and health care services for their people.

There is a change in the medical behavior of the Navajo today. Western medicine is accepted. However, the Navajo still believes strongly in his own religion, and rituals and medicine are still closely intertwined. The Singer and Hand Trembler are still very much a part of the health cure. When this does not work, scientific medicine is another means of treatment. There is a change also in that the Singer or Hand Trembler may suggest the patient go to the clinic or hospital. It must be recognized that religious rituals have a strong therapeutic effect and there is great support gained by the presence of all the family and friends who gather to help. The health professional needs to understand and accept this mixture.

In this author's small study, five humorous incidents involving the Indian were reported. Three of these reflected the minority feelings and the teasing of the white man.

> When the Indian patient was asked about his name "Limpy," he proceeded to tell the story of his great-grandfather who fought at the Little Big Horn massacre and was given the name Limpy by his ancestors when he wounded a white man causing him to limp!
>
> Another Indian patient with a scar on his back made jokes about "being knifed in the back."
>
> The third incident occurred between a Crow Indian nurse's aide and a white patient. The aide had entered the room with another aide who was Filipino. The patient teasingly asked if there were any Americans around. The Indian aide responded with, "What do you mean? I'm the first American!"
>
> In the fourth incident, the patient was a Kickapoo Indian who upon being told that the tumor she had was not malignant, sighed with relief and said "I thought I had swallowed a snake." The nurse reacted with surprise rather than laughter and the patient had to say, "That's a joke!"

Although the nurse did not pursue this "joke," we might speculate on its significance to the culture. According to the Indian culture, snakes are realistically feared, but are to be avoided rather than killed. It is a taboo to kill many creatures. Eating them is definitely a taboo. The patient may have been making a joke about the superstitious belief that violation of a taboo had caused her illness. However, the nurse did not understand this, and therefore did not "get the joke."

The fifth incident which involved a Kickapoo Indian child playing hide and seek with the School Nurse each time she was to receive her medication, appeared to be typical child's play.

These examples, as small as they are, reflect the admixture of old culture and new.

Spanish-American Culture

Anthropological studies and literature on the use of humor in the Spanish-American culture are nonexistent. More literature is available describing the relationship of the culture to health and illness. References to joking and teasing as a way to indoctrinate the young into the culture, in family relationships, and in peer relationships, are alluded to indirectly in a study by Madsen.[10] Much kidding and joking among males occurs as a way to show respect for courage, for "machismo," and for being a "true man," that is, to drink more, to defend himself better, and to be more virile than any other man. The male is jokingly compared to a rooster. The woman, on the other hand, is to be submissive, weak, and "pure." A loose woman is often the object of jest and ridicule. One might expect that a woman in this culture rarely teases or jokes with the man.

Humor also serves as a leveling mechanism. Achievements, better position, more wealth, create envy which is considered a destructive emotion. Therefore, one must not flaunt his success, rather he should play down his achievements, or others will do so through teasing.

Pedro, who came into the Catino dressed in a new suit, was teased about "running for mayor." "Pedro has come into money. The drinks are on him."[11]

Joking is also used as a way to solidify the cohesiveness of the culture, ridiculing Anglo behavior, implying it is good to be Mexican.

The written humor or comedy has generally come out of Mexico, South America, or Cuba. Comic books are read extensively by the masses in Mexico, and are used as a means of social commentary and political satire. A poster of cartoons in Spanish, *Chistes,* published by the Spanish Poster Service of Homestead, Florida, reflects both the American culture and the Spanish. One cartoon shows a family portrait in color in which all the family is white with one fellow dressed in black with long black hair, mustache and beard. The caption is *Oveja Negra* (the Black Sheep). It conveys several messages. One is the incongruity of applying the term "black sheep" to humans in a family portrait. But the changing values and attitudes are also conveyed: the move from being "white" and fair in color, which has been an admired characteristic in Spanish and Latin American countries, to the new generation's respect for being dark-skinned. The new Chicano often calls himself *Brown.*

The cultural beliefs of the Spanish-American around health and illness have been well described. These beliefs are in many ways similar to those of the Navajo. Religion, rituals, folk medicine and curing, and the belief that man has only limited control over nature are similarities that greatly affect the response to illness and health care.

The Spanish-American views himself as a passive victim of malevolent forces in his environment. God gives health and also sends illness. The illness may be viewed as a punishment from God or as a cross to bear. One patient believed he was paralyzed by polio because he kicked at his mother. Other illnesses may be caused by witchcraft or by careless or malicious behavior of others. Therefore, one is not to be blamed for being ill because of a personal lack of care or neglect.

Mal ojo or *evil eye* is an illness (usually in children) that is caused by someone admiring the child to an excessive degree. The prevention or cure is to have that person touch the admired or afflicted one. *Empacho* is a condition in which contaminated food is given to an individual because of maliciousness, while *mal de susto (illness of fright)* is caused by some emotional and frightening experience. *Maleficio* (or witchcraft) can be caused by malicious friends or witches. Some witches produce pain by forcing an evil wind (*mal aire*) to enter a victim's body. Prayers, ritual acts, folk medicine, and folk practitioners are used in the treatment of these illnesses. The *curandero, medico, sobador,* or *albolario* are used to diagnose as well as treat.

There is little emphasis on illness in the future; rather, illness is viewed as being in the present. Therefore, preventative practices, like immunizations, are not viewed with the same concern as the health professional views them. Keeping the mind and body in balance in order to be healthy, however, is important. The balances of "hot" and "cold" in relation to the body, to foods, and to interpersonal relationships are well defined.

The family is also an important consideration in making decisions and in giving support during times of illness. The patient does not deal with illness alone. The Spanish-American, therefore, expects that the curer or health professional will be warm and friendly and interested in all aspects of his life, as the *curandero* and his family are. The therapist must not be too impersonal and clinical. And, above all, he must not laugh at or ridicule the patient's beliefs. As with the Navajos, changes in medical beliefs and scientific medical practice have been accepted, but there is a mixture of both that must be recognized by the professional.

Some of these beliefs and attitudes are reflected in the humorous incidents reported and the opinions expressed by the health personnel in the study. One of the Mexican-

American nurses felt that one must be careful in using humor with the Spanish-American because it may be taken seriously, especially if it indicates any kind of blame. Illness is often regarded as a form of punishment. Joking, she found, was used mainly as a denial of illness and of its seriousness. But once accepted, the laughter often turned to tears. This is the reason many patients do not come to the clinic until very seriously ill. She gave several examples:

A young adolescent girl with a lump in her breast joked about having only one breast and what her boyfriend would do.

A male patient with a bleeding ulcer joked about getting drunk and eating too much chili; if the nurse would come and cook for him, he would be fine.

Another cardiac patient who had been put on a regimen of restricted activity and diet following surgery, was brought in from a bar where he had collapsed. He joked about having to drink to keep up his "machismo," and teased the nurse about coming home to take care of him.

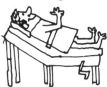

The husband of a patient who had cancer of the cervix had initially refused to let his wife go to the hospital, wanting more children, afraid his wife was not "going to be a woman." He joked with the nurse in a flirtatious way about being a woman. The nurse related that she had had a hysterectomy and asked if she "was less than a woman, now."

Several other examples from the study have to do with male manliness and male-female relationships:

A 14-year-old adolescent male was given a pre-football physical examination by the nurse practitioner. When she asked him to lower his shorts so that she could check for a hernia, he hesitated, and then asked if the other boys had allowed her to do this. Finally he said, "Well, it's okay but I'm not going to look!"

Another older Spanish-American male patient teased the male aide who was removing his cast about not getting too close to certain parts of his body.

Another Spanish-American male patient who was recovering from knee-cartilage surgery was asked by the Spanish-American nurse's aide how he was doing. He laughed and said, "Not so good, I can't get my leg up to make love to my wife."

In pre- and post-interviews with the staff from the Spanish-American Clinic and other Spanish-American health personnel, the question was asked whether they felt there was a difference in the humor used by the culture if the professional was a nonmember of the culture. The responses varied from *no difference* to *yes.*

One professional, a White, said she had heard the same Polack joke in South America that she heard in Wisconsin, except that the local minority group in that country had been substituted for Polack: "Where would you hide money from a Polack? Under a cake of soap."

The Mexican-American nurse, on the other hand, felt there was a difference if the professional was a nonmember, particularly in male-female interaction. The Spanish-American male may joke with her, but such behavior from an Anglo may be misinterpreted and taken seriously. She gave an example:

A young Anglo laboratory technician was very solicitous of a young Spanish-American male who had been brought in with an overdose of drugs, and teased him as he was recovering. The patient became very upset when she subsequently rejected his request to take her out.

In a discussion of cultural beliefs, the head nurse, who was white, said, "You know, I may have innocently put the *mal ojo* on babies and children, because I didn't know." One of the Chicano staff laughed and said, "Oh, we know how stupid Anglos are, so it doesn't bother us."

The implications from this discussion are that there must be trust and respect before humor will be understood and acceptable. Even a Spanish professional must know the patient well. In the case of a nonmember this relationship is even more crucial.

Black-American Culture

In reviewing the literature of the Black-American culture, humor has been integrated into all the other issues surrounding the history of the Black man in this country, and reflects the changes which have occurred. The original anthropological studies describing the joking relationship were observed in African tribes. Africa is the origin of the Black-Americans of today. However, the humor patterns of that culture could hardly be transposed to the new culture and circumstances in which the black slave found himself on these shores, since the situation and the relationships determine a joke culture. Perhaps the one aspect that has remained is the ability to laugh at harsh reality and tragedy. Anthropologist Laura Bohannan in her classic novel (under the *nom de plume* of Eleanore Smith Bowen) which relates the life of an anthropologist doing field work with a primitive tribe in Nigeria, describes this quality.

> They knew how to live at close quarters with tragedy, how to live with their own failure and yet laugh. . . . Such laughter has little concern with what is funny. It is often bitter and sometimes a little mad, for it is the laugh under the mask of tragedy, and also the laughter that masks tears. They are the same. It is the laughter of people who value love and friendship and plenty, who have lived with terror and death and hate.
>
> To be worst,
> The lowest and most dejected thing of fortune,
> Stands still in esperance, lives not in fear;
> The lamentable change is from the best,
> The worst returns to laughter.[12]

During the period of slavery, the black man learned that self-deprecating humor accommodated his master and was not offensive. It became a subtle way of ridiculing white concepts of black stereotypes: verbal difficulties, chicken stealing, fighting, freedom from sexual inhibitions, laziness, dishonesty. The Negro preacher and religious practices were also the butt of such humor. The use of humor as a technique in racial conflict has been described earlier. Since the Blacks were the first minority group to force Americans to deal with the issue of racial prejudice, the humor of the Black revolved in large measure around this issue. The humor became overt rather than covert, and anti-White jokes became more aggressive.

Particularly enjoyable to the Black is any incident or joke which shows Jim-Crow backfiring. The situations in which the Black is treated as a "darky" and then discovered to be the superior of the White in distinction, rank, or education are common. Some humor has a macabre flavor. The story is told of a black college president stepping off a train, who puts his arms out to catch a white woman behind him who has tripped. He suddenly realizes he is in Atlanta, drops his arms, and lets her fall. A study of jokes among university students, comparing a Southern White University with a Negro University in 1959, found that the Negro students told four times as many anti-Negro jokes as anti-White jokes.

The humor of today, post-civil-rights movement, still shows a need by Blacks to express hostility toward Whites and to satirize themselves and their situation, but there is more openness and the humor is understood and enjoyed by the white man as well. The current literature describing the history and culture of the Blacks, the discrimination, and the problems, along with courses on Black studies, have assisted in this understanding and change.

In the literature on health and illness in the Black-American culture, one early study of culture influences on patient behavior describes the use of humor by black patients in a southern hospital.[13] Most of the patients were of low income status and poorly educated and did not seek medical care early. A lack of understanding of their illness was evident and they were obviously hesitant to ask for service or express dissatisfaction. One method attempted was through joking and humorous behavior. The problem was that the nursing staff missed the cues because they either resented it or did not understand the function of the behavior and only looked at it as "cute."

There is an element of suspiciousness and lack of trust on the part of the black patient which keeps him from using health care facilities until he is quite ill. He fears the prejudice, impersonality, and bureaucratization. The history of the health status of the Negro is directly related to his social status and social relations. As his status improved and his educational, economic and social activities increased, so did his health status improve. In the past 60 years there has been a change from magical medicine to acceptance of the concept of disease and scientific medicine, although elements still remain. Many Blacks still seek as a first recourse the lay referral system: that is, pseudo- and para-medical healers, the fortune-tellers, mediums, herbalists, and makers of home remedies. Lack of funds and lack of sophistication with the health care system prevent many from seeking care. Preventive medicine for many is nonexistent, not from lack of awareness, but rather related to the general concept of future orientation. The body is just another object to be worn out and not repaired, to be enjoyed in youth and suffered and endured in old age. This concept changes as the Black becomes more middle class. For the many deeply religious Blacks, there is also an element of perceiving illness as a punishment. Therefore one puts oneself in the hands of God and asks the minister to pray, rather than seeking medical care.

Leininger describes two situations in the care of the

Afro-American patient. In one case, the black Southern male had difficulty trusting that the white nurse was really interested in caring for him since help and care given to the black people by the Southern whites is not common, especially by someone in a superior position. In the second situation, a black nurse who had been born and reared in the north, was uncomfortable taking care of a black male patient from the South. She noticed his mannerisms and language were different from hers and she did not want to be identified with these behaviors.

As with the Indian and Spanish-American cultures, there are variations in the black culture throughout the country and between various economic and status levels. Many patients resist seeking medical care because of the lack of understanding of differences in the diseases which affect them and the differences in care required.

In the study conducted by this author, many of these points were evidenced. One black professional, in an interview, felt Blacks use humor both to express hostility and to deal with the stresses. Some jokes with racial overtones, she said, can be shared with other minorities, but not with Whites, and many jokes which would be denigrating if initiated by Whites are tolerated within minority groups. Because of the cultural paranoia, she felt most Blacks would be suspicious of any joke initiated by a White, especially anything which might reflect stereotypes.

That Blacks do joke with each other about White stereotypes of them was described by one black aide with this joke:

A black man who had been walking stopped outside a White mortuary. He was tired and asked if he could rest inside. He laid down on a table in a room with two dead bodies and fell asleep. The embalmer comes in and rolls all three tables into the embalming room. Later, he comes out and tells the boss all three bodies are done. The boss tells him there was only two! The embalmer replies: "There were three, two white and one black." The boss says, "But the black man wasn't dead!" The embalmer says, "You know, he kept trying to tell me that. But, then, you know how those Blacks lie!"

However, these "anti-Negro" jokes which satirize the stereotypes would not be told to the white man, this aide contended, because Blacks would never "put down" the black man in front of the white man; rather the humor used would get back at "Whitey." There are many jokes, she said, that are told in the black community that would be reversed so that the white man is the butt of the joke when told to a white man.

Some of this is changing, and in an atmosphere of trust and acceptance, the humor around racial differences can occur. Two examples of humorous incidents described by a white nurse in this study points this out.

A young black male, waiting impatiently in the clinic to see the physician, joking with the nurse about not having to go through all that jive about checking in, said, "You know they call me J.J. [referring to the TV character in the show *Good Times*]. I'm just like him." The nurse laughed and said, "You're better looking than J.J., but just as ornery!" The patient continued to mimic "J.J.s" manner of walking and talking, apparently enjoying the situation.

Another black male patient, bundled to the ears in heavy coat, scarf, gloves, hat, and ear muffs, on a cold wintery day, began to slowly take off one piece at a time as he searched for his hospital plate to give to the clinic clerk. The nurse said, "You look awfully cold this morning." He said, "How can you tell?" She responded, "Cause your nose is red!" The patient laughed and all the other patients waiting behind him roared also.

Another example was reported by a white nurse caring for a black male patient following lung surgery. The patient was complaining about coughing all night and jokingly said he "thought he was coughing up sutures. Black, of course."

There were the same varied responses from the professionals when questioned as to whether there was a difference if the professional were a nonmember of that culture. Some said there was no difference, and several of the humorous incidents reported showed a good relationship but could have occurred in any nurse-patient interaction. However, there were those who felt there was a difference. The black culture has a language of its own, one nurse said, both literally and figuratively. Persons from the same culture can interact with each other in a soft joking way with language that would sound hostile if used by whites.

> A black male patient waiting in the clinic to see the physician was complaining loudly, "I've been here two hours!" The black nurse's aide smiled and said, "I've been here four hours. What you complainin' about?" The patient laughed and settled down again to wait.

Although not related to health and illness per se, a recent book by an educator, describing the problem of educating minority group, lower economic level youngsters in our inner cities, may serve to illustrate how an understanding of the culture makes a difference.

The youngsters used their streetcorner behavior to test their new, well-intentioned, middle-class teacher. Pupils walked in and out of the room, asking about reading comics, and getting off last period. Someone threw a crumpled-up piece of paper at the teacher. Thinking about his psychology courses which said, *Decontaminate through humor; make a joke out of things,* the teacher said, "If that's the best you can do, you'd better hang it up!" Whereupon "all hell broke loose." The class set out to show him they could do better.[16]

The humor failed because the teacher did not understand that, in streetcorner behavior, one must always prove one's self physically, without a show of fear. It is a life style that courts violence and physical aggression. His pupils expected the same from him. Even black parents expect teachers to be tough disciplinarians and "make" their children learn. They view fear as prejudice!

When the teacher began to understand the culture and the language, his style of humor changed and was effective. The students understood extroverted outgoing humor. "Acting crazy," "woofing," and "ribbing" helped: such behavior as hanging one youngster on a hook on the classroom door or jumping on the desk in "impassioned presentation." Often, the teacher would pick up a paper and read, "Wow — did you see this? John Frank was picked up by the police outside of the A&P on 125th Street for stealing a lollipop from a baby in a carriage." As the class laughed and howled, the teacher would note who was laughing the loudest and go on reading, inserting that youngster's name, "Jose Rodriquez was arrested for knocking over a Boy Scout helping an 80-year-old lady across the street."[17]

Humor, to be effective, not only requires an acceptance and understanding of the cultural background, but also requires an atmosphere in which humor is acceptable and in which there is mutual trust and respect for each other. Of the total 29 humorous incidents, both observed and past recollections, 17 emanated from one unit, the surgical Outpatient Clinic of a large general hospital. This seemed to be the direct result of the atmosphere of that unit. The head nurse used humor with both patients and staff as a normal part of her interaction. She felt it was the only way she kept the staff able to cope with a hectic daily schedule of an average of 180 patients a day, often with some 20 physicians coming in and out. She used humor to control the situation, to give direction. When she needed to correct or admonish someone she used "pet names" which set the frame for knowing "something was coming." When Albertine, the black desk clerk, became loud and noisy, the nurse would say, "OK, Albertooney..." or "Razzevelt" for the black orderly, Roosevelt. If the staff were madly dashing around, she might say, in passing, "If you're confused, maybe you need hormones!"

Since it was an inner city hospital, the patients who used this clinic came from all ethnic groups and cultures. The staff was also mixed. The head nurse was white, with three white, three black, and three Chicano staff. The head nurse felt that having staff of varied cultures was a distinct advantage in meeting their patients' needs. Very often "they can respond to each other in a language of their own."

In her interaction with patients, she had very carefully thought through her philosophy. "There needs to be respect and compassion and concern for the patient to use humor. The patient has to trust you and although sometimes the humor is rank, and you need to be direct and honest, you never make fun of or put the patient down. You catch his sense of humor!" She used humor to ease situations, but always came back to "concern."

> Many patients who come to the Clinic are elderly, economically in poor straits, often on fixed incomes. Yet, the hospital screening process requires that each time the patient must be asked if there is any change in income. The head nurse often says: "You haven't married a rich man since last time?" or "Found an oil well?" Then perhaps something like: "I know how hard it must be to manage today with this inflation."
>
> In teaching post-cast care to a patient with an extensive leg cast, she explains how to manipulate with it and then says "Wait till you try to sit on the john!" This always gets a laugh! Then she goes on to explain how to support the leg when sitting.

Sometimes, one must be alert to cues given by the patient that he is using humor to ease a situation.

> A chronic alcoholic with severe brain damage, during the screening process, had obvious difficulty with his speech and thinking. He could not seem to respond to a question regarding his address. An alphabet kept coming out rather than numbers. The nurse finally just moved on to the next question. "Nationality?" The patient smiled and said, "Well, I'm Polack." Both patient and nurse laughed.

The head nurse also gave an example of her humor that failed.

> An 80-year-old woman, with bleached blond hair, who always gave her age as somewhere between 47-55, consistently came in without an appointment and always wanted to be seen immediately. The nurse jokingly said, "Anyone as beautiful as you should be seen." The patient did not smile, rather she reacted negatively to the humor.

The humor hit too close to home: her obvious denial of reality, of her age and loss of beauty. There is always that fine line when teasing may become an insult.

CONCLUSIONS

There is much more investigation and research to be done in this area. The results of this study cannot give us conclusive answers to the questions we have raised about humor and culture. Perhaps it has only raised more questions! When we describe a culture, are we accurately portraying a people? Or are we portraying a stereotype? Are we describing characteristics which are a function of being poor rather than ethnic characteristics? What really constitutes an "American?"

The diversity of opinions expressed in this study suggests that there is a diversity within each culture or ethnic group, not only group or geographic differences but individual differences as well.

Therefore, the first basic assumption is that the cultural background of the patient must always be a consideration. The second assumption is that each person must then be assessed in terms of where he is within that culture. Here, a knowledge and understanding of that specific culture will be helpful in making this determination. The patient's degree of acculturation into Western culture must be evaluated. The Navajo from the reservation, the Chicano from the barrio, the Black from the ghetto have a different perspective compared to his counterpart who has attained middle- and upper-class status and a university education.

Most important to remember is that within all cultures there are changes in attitude. No longer do we find embarrassment or rejection, but rather a resurgence of pride in an ethnic heritage. Expression of this feeling ranges from a quiet display to an aggressive overreaction. Most individuals are simply incorporating the old and the new into a more comfortable way of life.

Just as the humor of a group or culture gives us clues to the function of that group, so the humor of each individual will reflect where he is in relation to his culture. And, of course, the degree of trust and respect and friendship established between patient and health professional will always make a difference in the degree and kind of humorous exchange which is acceptable.

REFERENCES

1. Leininger M: *Nursing and Anthropology: Two Worlds To Blend.* New York, John Wiley and Sons, 1970, p 45.
2. *Ibid,* p vii.
3. Radcliffe-Brown AR: On joking relationships. *Structure and Function in Primitive Society.* New York, The Free Press, 1952, p 90.
4. *Ibid,* p 91.
5. Mikes, *Laughing Matter,* p 115.
6. Myrdal G: *An American Dilemma.* New York, Harper, 1944, pp 38-39.
7. Burma JH: Humor as a technique in race conflict. *Am Soc Review* 11:710-715, 1946.
8. Hill WW: *Navaho Humor.* General Series in Anthropology, No. 9. Menasha, Wisconsin, George Banta Publishing Co, 1943, p 7.
9. Deloria V Jr: Indian humor. *Custer Died For Your Sins.* New York, MacMillan Co, 1969, pp 146-167.
10. Madsen W: *The Mexican-American of South Texas.* New York, Holt, Rinehart and Winston, Inc, 1964.
11. *Ibid,* p 23.

12. Bowen ES: *Return to Laughter.* The Natural History Library. New York, Anchor Books, Doubleday and Co, 1964, p 297.
13. McCabe GS: Cultural influences on patient behavior. *Am J Nurs* 60:1101-1104, August 1960.
14. Leininger, *Two Worlds To Blend,* 104-106.
15. *Ibid,* p 94-95.
16. Foster HL: *Ribbin', Jivin', and Playin' The Dozens, the Unrecognized Dilemma of Inner City Schools.* Cambridge, Mass, Ballenger Publishing Co, 1974, p 8.
17. *Ibid,* p 254.

ADDITIONAL BIBLIOGRAPHY

Adair J, Denschle KW: *The People's Health, Medicine and Anthropology in a Navajo Community.* New York, Appleton-Century-Crofts, 1970.
Flugel JC: Humor and laughter. *In* Lindsey G (ed): *Handbook of Social Psychology.* Cambridge, Mass, Addison-Wesley, 1954, pp 709-734.
Grotjahn M: *Beyond Laughter,* p 196-197.
Hines RH: Health Status of Black Americans. *In* Jaco EG (ed): *Patients, Physicians and Illness,* 2nd ed. New York, The Free Press, 1972, pp 40-50.
Kluckholn C, Leighton DC: *The Navajo.* Cambridge, Mass, Harvard Press, 1946. Natural History Library Revised Edition, 1962.
Leighton A, Leighton DC: *The Navajo Door.* Cambridge, Mass, Harvard Press, 1944.
Levine J: Regression in primitive clowning. *Psychoanalytic Quarterly* 30:72-83, 1961.
Levine J: Humor. *In* Sills D (ed): *International Encyclopedia of the Social Sciences.* New York, The Macmillan Co, 1968, pp 1-7.
Middleton R, Moland J: Humor in Negro and White subcultures: a study of jokes among university students. *Am Soc Review* 24:61-69, February 1959.
Nava J: Foreword. *In* Wagner NN, Haug MJ (eds): *Chicanos: Social and Psychological Perspectives.* Saint Louis, CV Mosby, 1971, pp xxi-xxiii.
Reichard G: *Navajo Religion.* New York, Bolligen Foundation, 1950.
Simmons D: Protest humor: folkloristic reaction to prejudice. *Am J Psychiatry* 120:567-570, December 1963.
Steiner S: *The New Indians.* New York, Harper and Row Publishers, 1968.
Thompson S: The trickster cycle. *The Folktale.* New York, The Dryden Press, 1946, pp 319-328.

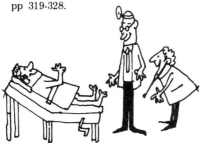

cultivating the use 3 of humor

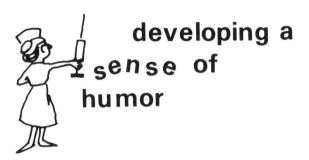

developing a sense of humor

We have been emphasizing the value of humor. We have shown that it is a form of communication which permeates our whole society, including the world of the health professional. We have also repeatedly voiced the opinion that not only must humor be understood, it also should be used as a deliberate therapeutic tool.

But how does one go about learning how to use humor consciously and effectively? Does that mean becoming a quipster? Building a repertoire of jokes? Becoming a clown? A practical jokester?

> I enjoy humor, but I've never been a joketeller, I can't even remember a joke.
>
> People say I'm funny, but I don't know why they laugh!
>
> Don't you have to be born with a sense of humor? You either have it or you don't!

These are typical reactions. The answer to all these questions is *yes* and *no! No*, because we should do only that which is comfortable for ourselves, that which suits our particular personalities, and fits our particular styles. Even a smile or a simple pleasantry can open doors and seem to create miracles.

And *yes*, because like any other skill or technique humor can be cultivated and learned. There are many suggestions and techniques which can be learned and, with practice, become an integral part of one's pattern of communication.

> We regard the humorist, like the poet, as born, and not made, but this isn't quite true. Humor can be cultivated. It is made up of confidence, independence, boldness and observation.[1]

However, just reading a book on humor, or reading humorous material, or the determination to practice humor is not enough. Nor is a series of devices for creating one-liners or jokes enough, in itself, although all of these are helpful in producing the end product. Rather, the first necessary step is to evaluate ourselves, and our own "sense of humor." Humor is first and foremost an attitude — almost an attitude toward life, a willingness to accept life and to accept ourselves "with a shrug and a smile," with a certain lightheartedness.

> To accept, in the end, existence, not because it's wonderful, not because it's divine, not because it's just or reasonable, or even satisfactory, but simply and plainly because it's all we've got.[2]

Yet this is not a sense of resignation or even indifference, but rather a sense of mastery over life. D.H. Monro has called this a "god's-eye view." It implies the ability to be objective, to view the absurdity of one's plight and to be a free, detached observer of one's fate.

A precise definition of a "sense of humor" has never really been attempted. It usually includes this readiness and ability to laugh at ourselves, our own weaknesses, and to grant ourselves a degree of humanness, but it also implies an appreciation of humor as well as an ability to create humor and to "be funny." We often attribute a sense of humor to the person who is always laughing and smiling and "making jokes."

Eysenck refers to three different meanings to the sense of humor. If someone laughs at the same things as we do, that is the *conformist* meaning. If he laughs a great deal and is easily amused, that is the *quantitative* meaning. If he is the life of the party and tells funny stories and amuses others, that is the *productive* meaning.[3] What we will be referring to in our use of the term *sense of humor* is an attitude which encompasses all of these meanings or dimensions, an attitude which senses the ludicrous and the absurdity of life, and which can be expressed in a variety of ways.

How does this attitude come about? Is it an instinctive quality, one with which we are born? Or is it a developmental process? Actually, most studies indicate that it is laughter or the smile which is considered instinctive, and the sense of humor as we have defined it, a developmental process, one which follows the course of normal physical, social, intellectual and emotional development.

The smile is the first social response of the infant which phylogenetically evolved from the startle reflex and has developed in man into a pleasurable reaction to small and pleasant stimulus changes. Rene Spitz in his famous study showed that the baby must see the full face and both eyes of the mother in order to respond. When the mother turns away the smile disappears.[4] The implications are that the contact, cuddling, and playing by a mother fosters the smiling-laughter response. The earlier the smile, the earlier the laugh, and the more advanced the development. With his smile the infant establishes himself as a human and a social being. The inability to smile demonstrates emotional starvation and loss of human contact.

The smile of the infant develops into the laughter of the baby. Play activity between adult and child in this early period consists of gross motor activities like tickling, bouncing, tossing in the air, chasing, and peek-a-boo. The baby's first reaction is startle and surprise which quickly turns to broad smiles and shrieks of laughter. The laughter is an expression of pleasure in the physical contact as well as relief from the initial alarm. This same element of surprise remains in adult humor with the corresponding burst of laughter following the punch line.

When the child begins to talk, this gross motor humor gives way to verbal humor. Rhyming words and displacement of words that have to do with toilet functions and the genitals produce laughter in the two- to three-year-old. As he begins to master bodily movements — *i.e.,* walking, toilet-training and other coordinated activities — his laughter is a response of superiority to these anxiety-producing situations. He laughs at the clown's clumsiness and antics and at involuntary or imitated flatus. The "belly laugh," says Grotjahn, stands halfway between the socially accepted noise of laughter and certain toilet noises which are taboo in company.[5]

At four years of age, fantasy and imaginary playmates are characteristic of play, and humor is aroused by anything that is strange and unusual and "funny." The humor becomes silly and boisterous. There is name-exchanging and name-calling and wild laughter. There is a beginning interest in pictorial expressions of humor which show distorted figures or "funny" scenes and lead to an increased interest in "the comics."

At age five begins an interest in games, which indicates a playing together rather than the self-contained play of earlier years. The playing of cowboys and Indians, circus, house, cops and robbers consumes hours of time. This imaginative play combined with a beginning formalization of intellectual behavior produces the "riddle" as a pleasurable activity.

The riddle moves into the anecdotal joke at age six where there is a marked increase in verbal humor. The six-year-old suddenly develops a lusty interest in adult jokes and begins to develop a repertoire. Riddles and April-fool jokes and "moron" jokes are associated with a new interest in learning and with the issue of being smart or dumb. William Fry feels there is a transition at this age related to a beginning ability to abstract and conceptualize. This capacity is an essential ingredient in getting the point of a joke.[6]

From eight to ten years of age, the child makes attempts to create his own humor through practical jokes and punning. He may repeat "dirty jokes" which he does not always understand. The ten-year-old's jokes may not seem funny to adults but for him it is an attempt to play with ideas and words. This is also a period when there is a laughing at the misery and misfortunes of others, i.e., the fat man and the man who slips on a banana peel, an indication of an ego strong enough to disguise aggression in a socially acceptable way.

A more outward display of aggressive humor occurs in the pre-adolescent. Slapstick comedy, clowning around, poking fun, and hurling insults are the signs of a more direct use of aggression, but are consistent with the early rebellion against authority of the 10- to 14-year-old.

By 16, there is a more adult level of abstraction, and an understanding of subtle implications and double meanings in jokes and cartoons. There is an interest in how jokes are told: timing, wording, and skill. Real humor, some authors feel, does not appear until adolescence. The adolescent begins to develop a sympathy for others and his "laughing at" begins to decline. He can use humor positively to "kid" a friend or to respond to criticism with kidding. And, he attempts to create humor. When I asked my 16-year-old daughter to tell me a joke going around in her circle, she said "We don't tell jokes. We make them!" At a meeting of the youth group of the church, everyone who made a pun or witticism was finally fined five cents, so that the group could get on with the business at hand.

The development of a sense of humor thus parallels the development of the use of language and of thought, of the ability to reason and to conceptualize. Mature humor is the final integration of all the stages and signifies also an emotional maturity. The social, intellectual, and physiological tasks have been mastered. This mature humor is based upon deeper life experiences, and kindly, tolerant acceptance of oneself and therefore of others. A free and periodic regression to the enjoyment of the child-like humor of the comic, the clown, and slapstick comedy occurs and is possible because the energy is no longer needed for repression. The development of this mature or even "greater" humor described by McDougall, Freud and Maslow may go on long into adulthood.

What fosters the development of this sense of humor throughout childhood? The loving atmosphere in the home and school, freedom and opportunity to express oneself, and the experience of successfully coping with frustrating and anxiety-producing situations through humor are suggestions made by some authors. The modeling of the use of humor and frequent laughter by parents in the home is another consideration since children learn by imitation and identification. Much more research into these conditions for fostering humor is needed.

We can describe the normal, general course of the growth and development of a human being physically, socially, emotionally, and intellectually. Yet we know that each individual, based upon his experiences, develops his own unique combination of traits and characteristics, his own personality and behavior which sets him apart from everyone else in the world. Similarly, with the development of a sense of humor, each person develops his own distinctive pattern. What he finds funny, how he reacts to humorous situations, how he makes use of humor, as well as his ability to create humor and "be funny," may be quite different from the next person's.

There is the view also that personality and a sense of

humor are closely related and are not independent of each other. Goethe once said, "Men show their character in nothing more clearly than by what they think laughable."

Many studies, indeed, most experimental studies conducted by psychologists have focused on the relationship of personality to a sense of humor or humor preference. Again the evidence is not conclusive, but a summary of these studies may provide a beginning understanding of the complexity of the relationship.

Several early studies indicated that extroverts preferred orectic (aggressive and sexual) jokes while introverts preferred cognitive (complex-clever) jokes, and that extroverts prefer derisive, superiority humor while introverts preferred nonsense, fantasy types of humor. This indicates that a person's typical personality or behavior extends to his preference in humor.

Aggression seems to be one trait which has attracted much study. Perhaps this is so because of the difficulty many persons have in accepting the relationship. Two studies demonstrated that enjoyment of humor led to a decrease in aggressive feelings. However, another study, which contradicts the cathartic effect of aggressive humor, found that angry female subjects were more aggressive following aggressive humor.

Another research study questioned under what conditions one person's aggression toward another was judged to be funny. The investigators discovered that social perception was important. A good person's hostile act is seen as more humorous and less hostile. A victim who "deserves" the hostility he receives elicits more humor than an undeserving victim. O'Connell found that men appreciated hostile wit more than women, while women preferred nonsense humor. Byrne studied three groups of male neuropsychiatric patients and found that those who could express hostility either covertly or overtly found hostile humor more amusing than those who were unable to express hostility. Martin Grotjahn, discussing the sexual joke, suggests that the discharge of aggression through laughter may facilitate the free and joyful acceptance of sex.

Another aspect often studied is the relationship between humor and intelligence and creativity. Two authors found wit and comedy and creativity positively correlated. Singer and Berkowitz found the wit to be high on ideational creativity and the clown high on adaptive regression, but no relationship between wit and intelligence and no relationship between the appreciation of humor and the production of humor. O'Connell also found no correlation between appreciation of humor and ability to create humor. However, another study in 1971 found that highly creative children used an abundance of humor whereas college students lacked this relationship.

Several tests to determine personality factors and responses to humor have been devised over the years. The *Mirth Response Test*, based on Freudian theory, utilized cartoons as an instrument for probing personality and bringing out emotional problems. It was used on both normal and psychiatric patients. Other tests have used cartoons as a teaching device in classes on humor.

Mindess provides an informal test for the reader to discover his preference in humor.[7]

He utilizes jokes rather than cartoons and a five point rating scale. The jokes test four categories of humor: philosophical, nonsensical, hostile, and sexual. Examples are:

Love is a disease that creates its own antibody: marriage.
　　Very　　　　　　　　　　　　　　　　Not
　　funny　　　　　　　　　　　　　　　　funny
　　Q: What does a 300-pound canary say?
　　A: **CHURP!**
　　　Very　　　　　　　　　　　　　　　Not
　　　funny　　　　　　　　　　　　　　　funny

When two politicians accuse each other of lying, both of them are telling the truth.

Very   Not
funny   funny

A farmer is showing a beautiful lady visitor around his farm. They watch a bull lustily mating a cow. Putting his arms around the lady's waist, the farmer says "Boy, I'd sure like to do something like that." "Well, why don't you?" she replies. "It's your cow."

Very   Not
funny   funny

Mindess speaks to the rating problems which beset this kind of research in humor. Since our individual spontaneous humor varies from time to time and situation to situation, the moment of the testing may be reflective of our emotional state at the time. It is also difficult to compare a joke heard previously to a new joke. One joke may seem clever, but not laughable, whereas another moves the listener to laugh but is gross and not clever. What is important, however, is to note that we do indeed have a preference and that by pursuing this notion we can discover something interesting about ourselves.

If we have a clear-cut preference or a strong dislike for one type of humor, we should consider what this means in terms of our own dynamics. The implications are that if we prefer hostile humor, we are working off aggressive feelings. Whereas if we do not find hostile humor funny, we either have no resentful feelings or we are desperately afraid of showing how much anger we really have! The same line of reasoning applies to sexual humor. Those who prefer it need release from their impulses. Those who avoid it cannot accept that they have these impulses. Those who enjoy absurd or philosophical humor are touchy about emotions and are involved in thinking processes or enjoy toying with ideas and reason. Those who do not are not thinkers, but gut-reactors.

Weighing whether we laugh because we are

comfortable with that emotion or quality or because we have a problem with it, or, on the other hand, whether we do not laugh because it is no problem or too much of a problem creates some of the difficulty in analyzing the reaction scientifically. Other problems relate to the salience or relevancy of the topic. A single person who has no mother-in-law may not laugh at mother-in-law jokes. But he may laugh at the cleverness of the joke, even though he has no personal hostility toward mothers-in-law.

Most of us fall into the category of enjoying some of each type of humor and disliking some of each. It may be more realistic to make an ongoing analysis of our everyday reactions to humor and our own humorous creations. The spontaneous witticisms we come up with as well as our day-to-day reactions to our personal situations may be more revealing of our natural use of humor than formal tests. The importance of the information we obtain regarding our humor in relationship to our own personalities is to use it simply as a guide to our own sense of humor, being aware of the situation in which it occurs, the frame of mind we are in, and our emotional state at the time. If we gain some clue as to the general state of our sense of humor and a clue to the style of humor with which we are most comfortable in keeping with our individual personalities, we can then look to the obstacles blocking the further development of our humor and to the frame of reference in which our sense of humor needs to be cultivated and expanded.

Mindess provides us with some guidelines for expanding our sense of humor. So many restrictions have been placed on us as children in the process of growing up that, as adults, we are wrapped in our own security blanket and have lost the ability to be spontaneous and genuine. The spirit of disruption and the exhilaration which the baby feels as he flies through the air can be rediscovered if we let humor help us to escape from the ruts of our minds and our self-imposed prisons.

The first step to acquiring a lively sense of humor is a readiness to "slip loose from organized modes of being."[9] We must be willing to revel in utter foolishness, be impulsive, irreverent, and unashamedly childish. Laughter must be fed on awareness of the eternal human comedy. We must free ourselves from the bonds of conformity and "become elastic with regard to society's demands."[9] We should allow ourselves to challenge all the shibboleths by which we live and we will rediscover the exuberance we knew as children. This release through humor, however, must be brief and our conventional view of life must be repeatedly re-established so that we can enjoy release from it again and again.

Freedom from inferiority, freedom from morality, freedom from reason, from language, from naivete, from redundancy, from seriousness, and from egotism are other freedoms we must develop in expanding our sense of humor. We must foster the conditions which help us to become nonconformists whose motto is "nothing sacred," to dislodge our feelings of inferiority, modify our moral inhibitions, indulge in foolishness, break loose from habitual behavior, renew our playful spirits, and escape our inescapable conceit. Above all, Mindess says, the cultivation of humor requires that we learn to thrive on change.

None of these conditions is as easy to develop as they sound, because they conflict with our needs to be dignified, competent and superior creatures. However, if we believe that man has the capacity to change and to continue to learn and to change his behavior, then we must believe that man, even in adulthood, can continue to develop, cultivate, and change his sense of humor. If we could not so believe, then all educators and human behavior professionals should simply "fold up their tents and silently slip away." We *can* teach an old dog new tricks and we can cultivate a sense of humor!

What it boils down to, again, is that a sense of humor is an attitude — an attitude that allows us to see the absurdity in life, in events and situations, in others, and in ourselves. How we express this attitude becomes an individual matter. Some of us are a Bill Cosby, others of us are a Don Rickles, and some of us are a Gracie Allen. This attitude of being "in fun" as Eastman calls it, is the foundation or framework we must cultivate in ourselves as a base for learning comedy techniques, utilizing humorous material, and incorporating humor into our communication patterns.

REFERENCES

1. Hoffman WG: *In* Whiting P: *How to Speak and Write with Humor.* New York, McGraw Hill Co, 1969, p vii.
2. Mindess H: *Laughter and Liberation,* p 145.
3. Eysenck JH: Foreword. *In* Goldstein JH, McGhee PE (ed): *The Psychology of Humor.* pp xvi-xvii.
4. Spitz R: The smiling response: a contribution to the ontogenesis of social relations. *Genetic Psychology Monographs* 34:57-125, 1946.
5. Grotjahn, *Beyond Laughter,* p 75.
6. Fry, *Sweet Madness,* p 14.
7. Mindess, *Laughter and Liberation,* pp 176-178.
8. *Ibid,* p 23.
9. *Ibid,* p 41.

BIBLIOGRAPHY

Andrew RJ: The origin of facial expression. *Scientific American* 88-94, October, 1965.
Berkowitz L: Aggressive humor as a stimulus to aggressive responses. *J Pers Soc Psychol* 16:710-717, April 1970.
Byrne D: The relationship between humor and the expression of hostility. *J Abnorm & Soc Psychol* 53:84-89, 1955.
Eysenck HJ: The appreciation of humor: an experimental and theoretical study. *British J of Psychol* 32:295-309, 1942.
Eysenck HJ: *Dimensions of Personality.* London, Routledge, 1947.
Grotjahn M: Sexuality and humor — don't laugh. *Psychol Today:* 51-53, July, 1972.
Gutman J, Priest RF: When is aggression funny? *J Pers Soc Psychol* 12,1:60-65, 1969.
Harms E: The development of humor. *J Abnorm & Soc Psychol* 38:351-369, 1943.
Koestler A: *The Act of Creation.* 1964.
Landy D, Mattee D: Evaluation of an aggressor as a function of exposure to cartoon humor. *J Pers Soc Psychol* 121:66-71, 1969.
McGhee PE: Development of the humor response: a review of the literature. *Psychol Bulletin* 76:328-348, 1971.

O'Connell WE: The adaptive functions of wit and humor. *J Abnorm Soc Psychol* 61,2:263-270, 1960.

O'Connell WE: Creativity in humor. *J Soc Psychol* 78:237-241, 1969.

Pearson GA: A child's humor. *Nurs Sci* 3:95-108, April 1965.

Redlich FC; Levine J; Sohler TP: A mirth response test: preliminary report on a psycho-diagnostic technique utilizing dynamics of humor. *Am J Orthopsych* 21:717-734, 1957.

Schoel DR, Busse TV: Humor and creative abilities. *Psychol Rep* 29:34, 1971.

Singer DL: Aggression arousal, hostile humor, catharsis. *J Pers Soc Psychol* [8] (1,pt. 2):1-14, 1968.

Singer DL, Berkowitz L: Differing creativities in the wit and the clown. *Perceptual and Motor Skills* 35:3-6, 1972.

Smith EE, White HL: Wit, creativity and sarcasm. *J Appl Psychol* 49:131-134, April, 1965.

Wolfenstein M: *Children's Humor:* Glencoe, Ill, Free Press, 1954.

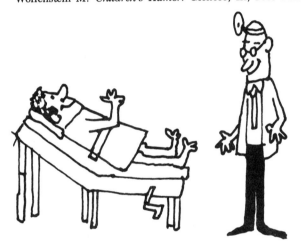

the
techniques
of
comedy

*Creating humor is
like asking how to
capture happiness.
It is elusive, sub-
jective, and inex-
plicable. You know
it when it's there
and you can feel its
absence.*

GENE REYNOLDS
Coproducer, *M*A*S*H*

How does one create humor? What makes it funny?
This has been one of the eternal questions surrounding
the concept of humor. Many theorists have responded as
Gene Reynolds did, for there is that quality of
uncertainty, intangibleness, and subtlety in humor.
William Fry refers to it as a "paradoxical abstraction."
We never really know if we have achieved the right
balance, the right nuance, the right spark, until we hear
that burst of laughter. Like happiness, the harder we try
to be funny, the more it escapes us.

Yet when pressed to define those elements, guidelines,
techniques which one pursues in producing comedy,
comedy writers are able to do so, as does Gene Reynolds
in describing the production of *M*A*S*H*.

> Comedy is lighter, smoother, more rhythmic than drama.
> One must avoid sobering assaults, long pauses, tight close-
> ups and strain...look for the smoothness, surprise, subtle
> gestures and the eccentric...and, above all, the
> recognizably human behavior must be painfully honest.
> When you can teach an actor the difference between
> playing dramatically angry and comically angry, you are
> warm.*

Excerpts from a personal letter, September 23, 1975.

Reynolds has described, very succinctly, the core elements in the creation of humor: the right timing, the smoothness, the subtlety, the surprise, the absurdity, and the human factor.

Humor which points out some very familiar human dilemma or weakness which "strikes home" will produce the laughter of recognition and acquiescence. Charlie Chaplin attributed his success in making people laugh to a knowledge and study of human nature. In his classic article on comedy, George Meredith conveys this same thought: "...to touch and kindle the mind through laughter demands, more than sprightliness, a most subtle delicacy."[1] The humorist must be "subtle to penetrate," and there must also exist a corresponding acuteness to welcome him.

> The life of comedy is in the idea. As with the singing of the skylark out of sight, you must love the bird to be attentive to the song, so...you must love pure comedy.... And to love comedy you must know the real world...[2]

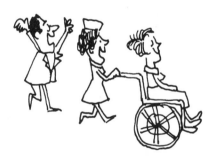

In more concrete terms, Sam Levinson suggests finding chuckles in the commonplace. Seek the common denominator in little things like television and dieting, and exaggerate it a bit. Robert Orben directs us to "think funny" and the comedy will "burst out in all directions."[3]

However, an attitude (which is what we are describing) must be practiced and developed if it is to become an integral, spontaneous aspect of our philosophy, view of life, and communication pattern. Furthermore, that practice must be a deliberate, conscious effort, often overpracticed and exaggerated, in order to be learned. There are a number of authors, joke writers and comedians who contend that humor can be cultivated and have described in detail how to create humor. Although their books are more in the realm of "how to" and for professional comedians, they nevertheless offer ideas for the would-be humorist in the health field. These guidelines for jokes, stand-up comedy routines, and one-liners may not always be appropriate for our own style of humor or for the quiet, simple pleasantries and situational humor which often occur in the health setting, but they do give us the essence of creating humor which is helpful in developing that quality of lightheartedness of "thinking funny," of the "god's eye view." In addition, they give us some tangible methods to practice, rather than just exhortations to "be funny," if we are to incorporate humor in a more calculated fashion in our communication patterns, in our teaching practices, and in interventions with patients.

THE BASIC ELEMENTS

Creating humor is somewhat like using a recipe to create bread: there are certain ingredients that must always be present if we are to achieve a recognizable product. However, there are modifications of these ingredients, and the addition of numerous other ingredients can create variations of the same product. There is also a distinctive pattern for blending the ingredients. There must be the right temperature and the right timing for cooking it. And, finally, the end result, to be fully appreciated and enjoyed, must be served in an appealing fashion to just the right audience.

So with humor to be effective there are two basic ingredients which must be present, with many variations and many other ingredients which can be added. Humor must be blended in just the right way, in the right atmosphere, with the right timing, and presented with elegance and smoothness to the right audience.

The two basic ingredients of humor which seem always to be present in some degree are surprise and absurdity. There must be some unexpected twist which creates a shock of surprise; that surprise must be absurd or ludicrous, yet fit into the general context of the story or concept. We must be led down one corridor of thought

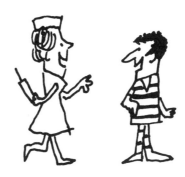

and suddenly jolted into another by some unexpected turn of events. There are many variations of this surprise and absurdity but, like flour and liquid, both are there in some form and to some degree.

The many modifications and additional ingredients are elements which include incongruity, contrast, conflict, misunderstandings, play on words, double meanings, allusions, exaggerations, overstatements, understatements, fantasy, and sheer nonsense.

Let us look at some examples. There is a cartoon of a man with an arrow through his chest leaning over the receptionist's desk in a doctor's office. The nurse looking at the appointment book, is saying, "How about a week from Tuesday?"

The surprise response and incongruity of the desperate patient and the casual nonchalant nurse is so absurd, we have to laugh! The cartoon also points out a familiar frustrating situation: having to wait to see the doctor. But the contrast here is so sharp, it is funny rather than annoying.

The humor must also "fit" to be amusing. If the nurse had simply said, "The doctor is not in," it would not have been humorous at all. The incongruity concept must be a sudden perception of two obviously incompatible ideas, meanings, emotions, objects, situations, or events.

The double-meaning ingredient can be shown by this story, attributed to Lewellyn Thompson, Ambassador to Russia in the Sixties.

> A Russian peasant is trudging down the road on a cold bitter morning when he sees a bird lying on the side of the road, half-frozen. In sympathy, he picks up the bird, holds it in his hands and tries to warm it. Spotting a freshly dropped, still warm pile of manure nearby, the peasant places the bird down in the middle of the pile, and goes on his way. Responding to the warmth, the bird gradually thaws out and feeling good, he begins to chirp and sing. A wolf, not far away, looking for his morning breakfast, hears the singing, comes trotting over, pounces upon the helpless bird who cannot extricate himself, and eats him.
>
> The moral of this story is, it is not always your enemies who put you in it, nor your friends who pull you out, but when you are up to your neck in it, for God's sake — don't sing!

We are led along with the story to a blank wall when the bird is eaten. So what's funny? Then, with a surprise twist, the story is turned into a moral with a double meaning attached. The absurdity, yet the direct "fit," of the moral makes us laugh.

Shaggy dog stories are another variation which are so unexpected and so nonsensical, they strike us as funny: "Why do you have that celery stuck behind your ear?" "Because I didn't have any lettuce."

A play on words — puns, mispronunciations, and malapropisms — create humor. They are surprising and ludicrous.

Archie Bunker consistently mispronounces words which, because of his air of superiority, becomes highly amusing. In a recent TV episode, he described to Edith how he had given a passenger in his cab mouth-to-mouth resuscitation and had taken her to the Intensive Care Unit of the hospital. In so doing, he calls it mouth-to-mouth "restitution" and the "expensive" care unit.

Exaggeration is an element dear to the heart of Americans and especially to Texans.

A fellow walks into a bar in Texas and orders a beer. The bartender places in front of him a huge 2-foot glass, and says, "Everything in Texas is big." As the stranger sits there drinking his beer, a tall Texas walks into the bar. The stranger gasps and asks, "How tall are you? "I'm 7'4″, replies the Texan, "everything in Texas is bigger." And, so it went. Finally, after all that beer, the stranger asks for direction to the rest room. He is told to go down the hall to the door on the left. However, in his state of inebriation, he opens the door on the right and falls into the swimming pool! He flounders and gasps, and as he is struggling to get to the side, he keeps yelling, 'DON'T FLUSH!!!'

The surprise ending, the ludicrousness of the situation, yet the obvious fit to the concept of "big" is vividly demonstrated.

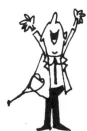

In addition to the basic ingredients, there must be a proper sequence and blending of those ingredients in order for the joke or humor to occur. The punch line must be held in abeyance and presented in such a way that the surprise is created and the point is made.

In a recent comic-strip, *The Family Circus,* one of the boys is reading a joke book. He says,

"Wanna hear a joke, Dolly?"
"Uh-huh!"
"Okay, how does a witch tell time?"
"I don't know — how?"
"She wears a WITCH WATCH!"

Dolly, gleefully, says, as she dashes off to the other room,

"I'm going to tell that one to Daddy!
"Daddy, do you know how a witch tells what time it is?"
"She looks at a clock, I suppose."
"No, she wears a watch on her wrist!"

Daddy does not laugh and looked perplexed, as Dolly runs off crying.

"Daddy didn't laugh at my joke!"

Dolly flubbed the punch line and the whole point of the joke was gone.

The proper sequence of events leading up to the punch line should also contain those points to which the punch line refers. The use of pauses, intonations, and gestures can also highlight the crucial points. A dialect should be used only if the individual can do so with finesse, but can add to the effect of the story.

Proper timing is essential to the success of humor. It must occur at just the right moment. Many a witticism in a discussion or conversation gets a louder laugh than the content itself would indicate, simply because it "fits" so well and strikes the right note. The pace or tempo is also crucial to the build-up of the suspense when a joke is being told. The punch line must catch the listener unaware — and ready — not lost in boredom along the way. Proper timing also implies an appropriateness to the situation; that is, the atmosphere must be conducive to that bit of levity.

To round out the basic elements of a humorous undertaking, the neatness or the "elegance" with which the sally is delivered is vital. The humor must flow smoothly. If the humorist stumbles, loses track, hems and haws, he has lost it. Sometimes a spontaneous witticism can save the occasion and is funnier than the planned story.

> At a recent national nursing conference, the Chairman of the meeting was telling a story and suddenly couldn't remember the punch line. The audience giggled as she hesitated, and said, "Oh dear, I've forgotten the punch line." Then, she recovered her composure and said, "You know, the brain is really a marvelous thing. It starts working the moment you awake in the morning, and only stops when you open your mouth in front of an audience."
> *That* brought down the house!

A little later when a friend reminded her of the punch line to her story and she relayed it to her audience, it was no longer funny. It was out of context, the timing was off, and the surprise element was gone.

Needless to say, the content of the humor is another crucial factor. Knowing your audience is the first prerequisite. Jokes about education to educators, about nursing to nurses, are more effective than those same jokes would be to business leaders or politicians. Even more specific, witticisms about education *per se* would not strike the fancy of the practicing staff nurse in the hospital, as it might the educator. However, humor about the current controversy that nursing educators are not preparing students for the "real world" of practice would hit home! Effectiveness, says Mindess, depends on the strength of the drive it releases in the listener. If it evokes a gut reaction, reduces anxiety, is not too gross and touches us where we live, it will be enjoyable.[4]

Max Eastman sums up the basic elements for serious joke-makers in his *Ten Commandments of the Comic Arts;* although the language is quaint, is still conveys the essence of our previous discussion.[5]

Commandments	Interpretation
Be interesting.	It must arouse an emotional interest.

Be unimpassioned.	Don't crack jokes around topics about which people feel too intensely.
Be effortless.	Don't try too hard to be funny.
Remember the difference between cracking practical jokes and conveying ludicrous impressions.	A practical joke is a witty joke, brief, with the fun in the punch line or the "nub," while a ludicrous impression is a humorous story which can be spun out and is amusing all the way through.
Be plausible.	Successfully lead the audience on.
Be sudden.	Save the punch line and make it a genuine surprise.
Be neat.	A joke with a point that gets across.
Be right with your timing.	It has to be sprung.
Give good measure of serious satisfaction.	Joke must amuse the audience.
Redeem all serious disappointments.	If the joke falls flat, redeem it by another funny comment.

STEPS TO BECOMING A HUMORIST

You are ready now to be a humorist, you say; where do you go from here? You have the right attitude, you understand the basic elements of a joke, now what?

Step One: Choose your weapon: your style.

Joey Adams suggests that we must choose our weapons, that is, find out what style is funny and comfortable for us. Do we see ourselves as a wit, a kidder, a humorous story teller, gag man, a joke-teller, a punster, a clown, a satirist, or a floater? Choose that comedy style, study that style, collect materials, and practice.

Each of these styles refers to a kind of humor. Generally, the average person enjoys and utilizes many varieties of humor, but some individuals, in keeping with their unique personalities, favor one variety over the other. If you find in your own analysis that one style seems to be your forte, recognize it and develop it. The descriptions of various styles provided in this book are adapted from Joey Adams' cookbook for humorists and are intended to give us clues in analyzing ourselves and clues to the variations in humor and style. The reader should compare these descriptions to well-known comedians and analyze his reactions to their styles.

A recent research study which investigated the relationships between different types of comedians and their audiences compared Bill Cosby and Don Rickles.[6] Cosby makes us laugh at bits of human behavior common to us all. He pokes fun at our fallacies, but is never hostile or confronts us directly. Rickles, on the other hand, picks on his audience, *Hello, dummy.* He makes fun of us and exposes our foibles. The subjects viewed Cosby as a nice guy, funny and harmless. They laughed at Rickles only if they were with a group of friends. Group solidarity was important: *I'll laugh, if you will.*

Comedy Styles*

The Wit: Thinks while he's talking. Transforms experience into humor; spins a humorous web of life and

---

*Adapted from Joey Adams.

expression. Makes use of the repartee, a witty, smart reply, a lightning retort. He is most respected because of this ability. Often the laugh is at the expense of others.

Satirist: The sword of wit, finds humor in controversial, social, political, and taboo issues.

Punster: Delights in play on words. Has a knack for puns, acronyms and mispronunciations. Is considered a simpler form of wit.

Clown: Overwhelms his audience with antics, little dialogue. Sees life as though reflected in fun-house mirror. Exaggerates, may use props and is expected to "clown around."

Joke-teller: Has a repertoire of jokes for every occasion. Relies on the buildup, the details, the dialect — not just the punch line. Believes it is the way the joke is told that counts.

Gag-man: New breed. He throws lines from any angle; the right joke at the right time for the right situation.

Humorous Story-teller: Pokes fun at daily happenings; is prepared with category of stories and jokes. He will settle for a smile or chuckle. The humor is more gentle and less aggressive. Often the humor is self-depreciating and relates his own dilemmas.

Kidder: Loves to tease. Jocular talk is part of his general pattern of communication.

Practical Joker: Plans tricks and jokes to play on others.

Do you see yourself in these descriptions? Or, do you see areas you would like to cultivate? Then move on to *Step Two.*

Step Two: Collecting materials — base line data.

Before we are ready to create on our own, developing a file of humorous materials will assist us not only in creating new jokes, but as an adjunct and resource base. Incorporating humorous material of others into our conversations, lectures, speeches, and writings is an effective tool which we should always use even when we find ourselves becoming more spontaneous and creative.

1. Make a file of jokes.
2. Jot down amusing anecdotes and humorous situations.
3. Listen for witty remarks others make.
4. Jot down humorous signs, TV gags.
5. Record personal humorous experiences.
6. Collect boners, and newspaper funnies.
7. Save cartoons and magazine humor.
8. Collect comedy records and humorous poems.
9. Collect materials of comedians and comedy writers.

Step Three: Creating your own humor.

The gimmicks and techniques which comedy writers use to create the humor they produce can be used by the new humorist. There are four approaches or methods:

1. Tell second-hand jokes or stories.
2. Share humorous experiences of your own and others.
3. Modify old jokes, quips, and stories.
4. Invent or create new humor by using humorous devices.

The first two approaches are self-explanatory and the techniques for the right timing, the appropriateness, and methods of delivery have been previously described. However, the gimmicks to practice for *three* and *four* are presented in outline form with examples attached.

A. *Devices for modifying old jokes, quips, stories, gags, quotations, etc.*

1. Switching: Dress up an old joke in new clothes. Joey Adams maintains there are seven original joke patterns: puns, insults, sex, domestic, underdog, incongruity, and topical (current topic or issue). Make these fit the situation.

"I don't fly on account of my religion — I'm a devout coward."

One frog says, "I've got a man in my throat."

"Old doctors never die — they just cut-out."

"Old psychiatric nurses never die — they go into administration."

"He who hesitates will hear horns tooting."

2. *Personalize and localize:* Substitute name of place, city, or person or group to whom you are telling the joke, story, or anecdote. Relate a joke as an actual incident involving someone well known to your audience.

A nursing leader discussing the discordancy and divisiveness in the profession, quipped, "What nursing needs is its own Henrietta Kissinger."

3. *Poke fun at yourself:* Audiences love to feel superior. Make jokes about things that are happening to you. Using yourself as the butt of the joke makes you human and endears you to your audience.

Following a "boo-boo" you've made: "Do you ever feel like you're in the wrong profession?"

B. Humorous devices for creating humor.

1. *The humorous catalogue:* The injection of a humorous item into an otherwise serious list.

"A politician on the campaign trail must be articulate, diplomatic, knowledgeable, have stamina and the digestion of an ostrich."

2. *Exaggeration:* So overstate a truth as to make it absurd, yet leave the original idea obvious.

"That room is so small, when you lie down the door knob gets in bed with you."

"My nursing instructor was so old, she didn't teach history, she remembered it."

3. *The double-cross:* Wreck a plausible train of

thought by an incongruous one and produce a shock of surprise.

> "He was determined to stay alive, even if he died in the attempt."

> "There once was a professor who dreamed he was lecturing and woke up to find it was true."

4. Anti-climax: A sentence or passage in which the ideas at the close fall off in dignity or importance.

> "Our next speaker needs no introduction. He didn't show up."

> "Now a quote from that famous child psychologist — our teenage babysitter."

5: The insult: Be sure of your gag and your audience.

> "Hello, dummy."

> Groucho Marx introducing a film: "Every once in a while Hollywood makes a great movie. Unfortunately, this isn't one of them."

6. Nonsense-fantasy-escape from reality: Gags are completely irrational and fantastically ridiculous.

> Dog 1. "I feel so poorly."
> Dog 2. "Have you thought of going to a psychiatrist?"
> Dog 1. "Heavens, no! You know I'm not allowed on couches."

7. Understatement:

> "If you can keep your head when all about you are losing theirs, maybe you don't understand the situation."

> Cartoon: Trapeze artist fails to catch his partner, says "Oops, sorry."

> Cartoon shows a fisherman in a rowboat on a lake, clutching a monstrous fish which is bigger than he is. Another man is rowing by and says "Had any luck?"

8. Irreverence: Poking fun at pomposities, lampooning authority and stuffed shirts.

> "He calls himself the Friendly Psychiatrist. He lies down on the couch with you. They call this socialized medicine."

> "The greatest obstacle to the advancement of medicine is atrophy of the ear."

9. *Invent topicals:* A humorous reference to some topic or issue of the day-headline news.

> President Ford: "I'm America's first instant president. The band is so confused, it doesn't know whether to play *Hail to the Chief* or *You've Come a Long Way, Baby.*"

10. *Humorous definitions:*

> "Adolescence is that period in a child's life when his parents become more difficult."

> "Area of expertise means you do everything else worse."

> "Statistics are like a bikini! What they reveal is interesting. What they conceal is vital!"

11. *Use "sight" laughs* with gimmicks.

> "The Chairman has asked me to say a few words." (Lifts a sheaf of papers three inches thick.)

> A sheet of paper attached to a new set of By-Laws reads: SEX. Now that I have your attention...please discard the old and read the new set of By-Laws.

12. *Deliberate mispronunciations, puns, use of abbreviations, acronyms:* Adds a brief but sudden jolt in a formal lecture or discussion, or conversation.

> "You're putting the emphasis on the wrong syl-la'ble."

> "That's a SWAG." (Scientific wild-assed guess.)

> Bill Cosby in TV show, *Feeling Good,* is a fertilized egg in a skit on prenatal care. He calls up to Mom to send down "some calcium and iron." When it clangs down, he responds with, "Thanks, that's real womb service."

SUMMARY

Now that you are hooked on humor, there are a few precautions and warnings from the old-timers. In your enthusiasm, don't try to be "too darned funny" or pile on too many jokes. Don't strain to add humor which doesn't fit the situation. Restraint is the keynote. Humor has a tendency, like anything else, to be destroyed by overuse. A few well-placed, well-timed funnies are much more effective. If you are giving a speech or a lecture, make your first story or joke a blockbuster. Everything after that will be funny. At least you will keep your audience awake waiting for the next one!

Never, never, tell a story or joke unless you like it yourself and really think it is funny. Not so funny that you are rolling in the aisles yourself. That will turn your audience off rather than on. But, because you enjoy it, you can give it the right tone. Practice it! When you tell a story, pause afterwards. Give your audience a chance to "get it."

Above all, "think funny." Look for chances to use humor, collect materials and practice! Analyze the humor you use. If it falls flat, why did it? Try again. Don't get discouraged and don't expect perfect results. Being humorous five per cent of the time is better than not being humorous at all. Once you try it, you may find you like it!

Humor is addictive!

REFERENCES

1. Meredith G: On comedy. *In* Felheim M (ed): *Comedy,* p 206.
2. *Ibid,* p 210.
3. Orben R: The Pied Piper of humor. *Talent,* Spring 1972.
4. Mindess, *Laughter and Liberation,* p 167-168.
5. Eastman M: *The Enjoyment of Laughter.* New York, Simon and Schuster, 1936, pp 290-326.
6. Murphy B, Pollio HR: I'll laugh if you will. *Psychology Today,* p 106-109, December 1973.

BIBLIOGRAPHY

Adams J: *Encyclopedia of Humor.* New York, The Bobbs-Merrill Co., 1968.
Harrel S: *When It's Laughter You're After.* Norman, Oklahoma, University of Oklahoma Press, 1962.
Orben R: *The Encyclopedia of One-Line Comedy.* New York, Doubleday and Co, 1971.
Whiting P: *How to Speak and Write With Humor.* New York, McGraw-Hill Co, 1969.

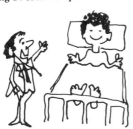

utilizing humor in communication, teaching and intervention: some beginning guidelines

'The time has come,' the Walrus said, 'To talk of many things: of shoes — and ships — and sealing-wax — of cabbages — and kings — and why the sea is boiling hot — and whether pigs have wings.

LEWIS CARROLL,
Through the Looking Glass

Indeed, the time has come! Not to talk of cabbage and kings, but to speak to the heart of the matter for which this book was conceived. We have consistently affirmed that humor is one of the most valuable tools a health professional can have. We have spoken to the *why;* we have spoken to the *what* and the *where* of humor. We have begun to speak of the *hows,* and now we are down to the last *how.* How do we apply this knowledge, this new ability to be witty and humorous? How do we use this humor to improve communication, facilitate teaching, and help our patients intervene in the stresses and the anxieties with which they must cope? This is the heart of the matter. If we could call upon the Gryphon's "Classical master, who taught Laughing and Grief," all our problems would be solved.

There are three major groups with whom we as professionals communicate: our colleagues, our students, and our patients. We tend to stereotype our roles with each of these groups, as friend, teacher, and health-care giver. It follows that we tend also to stereotype our functional utilization of humor for each of these as meeting sociological needs, educational needs, and psychological needs, respectively. This may be the foremost function of humor in each of these roles. However, in our usual communication patterns we find this is not always so clear-cut. Meeting sociological needs with our friends and colleagues, we sometimes meet their psychological and educational needs as well. With our students we are sometimes social and many times give psychological support. The same holds true with patients or clients. Our responses may be more in the direction of health teaching, and sometimes our communication is at a purely social level with no psychological overtones or directions. Guidelines for utilizing humor cut across roles, and, just as there is no content area which is not subject to humor, so there is no one discrete function for the use of humor within various categories of persons. Rather, it is the time and situation which are the determining factors. For convenience, however, in presenting the recommendations for the practice of humor, the three broad sections of the communication framework, teaching, and intervention have been developed. The overlaps will be obvious, but the need to operationalize these interactions for specificity is also indicated.

THE COMMUNICATION FRAMEWORK

Humor, we have said, is an indirect form of communication. Within health settings, it is apart from the "official normative system," and the choice to use humor is an optional matter. Because of the serious business of the hospital setting, Emerson expected to find in her study clearly defined areas and relationships where humor would or would not be used. She found instead that humor is permissible in almost any situation in the hospital and that humor is initiated by all categories of persons under almost any circumstances. This broad area includes colleagues, other staff, students, and patients. In only three instances did she find that humor did not occur: when patients were seriously threatening not to cooperate with staff, when the patient was extremely upset emotionally, and when the staff was interacting with the relatives or visitors of dying patients.

This freedom in the use of humor in actuality extends far beyond the hospital confines to other health agencies, to public health settings, to the home, to the classroom, and to society in general. However, within this freedom, if a choice to use humor is made, there are some informal social rules, and conventions or understandings about the initiation and conduct of humorous communication which must be considered.

Emerson has succinctly summarized the circumstances under which the choice to use humor in preference to other forms of indirect communication is made:

a) A humorous tone is appropriate in the situation. b) It is possible to introduce a playful note without disrupting the serious business. c) There is relatively more consensus and intimacy among the participants (as indicated, for example, by similarity in age, sex, and position in the organization) so that the chance of a misunderstanding about whether humor is intended is reduced. d) The actor is willing to take the risk that the message will be ignored. e) A relatively high degree of exemption from responsibility is desired. f) The actor has the social role of fool, or is personally expected to joke.[1]

In addition, in making a choice to use humor, the initiator must assess the receptivity of the other or others to his humor. Certain cues may indicate this acceptance: a previous joking relationship; ongoing humorous interaction; past or present initiations of humor by the other person; a feeling tone of receptivity as indicated by smiling, twinkling eyes, etc.; or a feeling of warmth, empathy and trust.

The initiator must also know his audience. He must evaluate whether the content will be understood, that the content will not be offensive, and that the message conveyed by the humor will be acceptable.

Once the decision to use humor is made, if it is to be successful, a framework must be established which is recognized by all concerned. The joke-frame says in effect: *This is a joke. It is in fun. It is not serious.* This joke-frame, says William Fry, is similar to a play-frame and is as vital to situation jokes as it is to canned or formal jokes or practical jokes.[2] The establishment of this joke-frame involves two basic rules or components.

The first rule is that the initiator must make it very clear that he is joking and that humor is his intent, particularly when it is initiated in a nonhumorous setting. The cues that humor is being initiated may be verbal or nonverbal. Verbal cues are actual statements such as "Let me tell you a story," "Have you heard this one?" "This'll kill 'ya." Most cues, however, are in the form of nonverbal metacommunications. They signal that there is a change in the interaction. The signal may be a gesture, a shift in posture, a change in facial expression or tone of voice. The person may smile, wink, or get a "twinkle in his eyes." His face may "light up." The tone of his voice may become lighter, teasing, or flippant. He may chuckle or giggle.

Sometimes, a dead-pan style of delivery, which is in direct contrast to these cues, may be used. In that context, the delivery is a joke in itself. It is generally used only when the relationship between the participants is such that it will be understood. That is, either this has occurred before in the relationship or the content of the humor is so obvious and so outrageous that it can only be assumed to be humorous. A sudden shift to dialect or to mispronounced words or distorted phrases or an obvious misinterpretation of a situation are examples of content which are enhanced by the dead-pan delivery.

The second rule in the joking framework is that the recipient of the joke must acknowledge the humor, unless he chooses to imply that the humor is inappropriate, at which time the joke-frame is dissolved and the humor is lost. A lack of response may also mean that the recipient did not understand the humor or failed to "get the joke." In the case of a patient who is lethargic or in pain, he may understand, perhaps even appreciate, the humor, but physically may be unable to respond. In either case, the joke-frame will not be set. The "license to joke" given by the recipient is usually acknowledged by a laugh or a smile. Sometimes, it may be a groan! A verbal response like, "You're funny, man!" or "That's a good one!" may occur. A counter-joke or humorous remark by the recipient may set up a continued banter or humorous exchange. Once a joke-frame is thus set or established, future encounters or joking relationships are likely to occur.

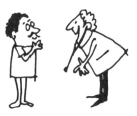

Two types of joking frames have been identified as occurring in social or cultural groups: *setting-specific* and *category-routinized.*[3] Essentially, the setting-specific implies that the joking activity revolves around specific persons and their identities in a particular setting. These joke-frames are short in duration and highly fragile, susceptible to disruption. Category-routinized are of longer duration and are less fragile because they revolve around known categories of persons and a certain routinized joking behavior. There is a high degree of consensus about the context of the joking and the content itself. Joke-frames may also be *contained,* that is, include only certain persons, or *uncontained,* that is, any member of the audience is free to participate.

The general communication framework for humor is applicable in any situation whether it be a one-to-one relationship or a group relationship, between staff and patient, between student and teacher, between colleagues or in setting the tone of a ward, a clinic, a classroom, or a professional conference. We will speak specifically to patient-staff interaction and to student-teacher interaction in the next sections, so an example from the same national nursing conference referred to previously might clarify this communication framework.

At a general session on the third morning of the conference, during a panel discussion, one of the panelists, representing a federal government agency, was speaking on the availability of federal funds to do what was needed in continuing education in nursing. She asked the audience to react spontaneously to what they saw as the future goals in continuing education and some of the needs to meet these goals. Several of the young leaders spoke to the lack of avenues for the preparation of identified potential leaders. Rather than a positive acknowledgment and acceptance of these individuals' personal ambitions and goals to be leaders, a condemnation of "smart-mouths" like themselves was often encountered. Getting to be a leader almost required a subtle denial of such ambition. As a result, the persons sometimes had the competency and sometimes not when they "fell into" the positions of leadership. Actual apprenticeships and internships with experts like the panelist was the solution these young persons from the audience were proposing.

The panelist acknowledged the need for leaders and

the need for legitimized avenues of preparation and then said, "but let me tell you a mythological story."

There is a $10,000 bill in the center of a conference table. At one corner of this table is sitting an Expert Administrator, at another corner is the Easter Bunny, at another corner is Santa Claus, and at the fourth corner is a Bumbling Administrator. Only one of the four can have the money. At the sound of the gong, who do you think got the $10,000 bill?

The answer is: The Bumbling Administrator, of course, because all the others are mythological figures!

There were many messages conveyed: *Don't put us on a pedestal. We're not perfect. Don't you expect to be perfect. There are no absolute experts. What makes one leader effective may be ineffective if tried by others.*

The humor used was very successful in this instance because the framework for communication through humor had been established. There had been many cues throughout that morning that humor was acceptable because both speakers and audience had made witty comments and there had been much laughter. The one young leader's reference to herself as a "smart-mouth" which got a big laugh, as well as other witty remarks, communicated to the panelist that she could also respond with humor. She also knew her audience and knew they were specific-centered enough to get the message conveyed by the joke without needing a serious lecture which would have been inappropriate at the time. Her self-depreciating joke also brought the tone of the meeting from a confrontation of "What have you not done for us and what are you going to do about it?" back to the original sharing, congenial atmosphere of what are *we* going to do about it.

PATIENT INTERVENTION

The humor used in the situation just described was very effective because the panelist had assessed the situation, knew her audience, and recognized that a humorous intervention would be appropriate. There was a subsequent reduction in tension and a return to social interaction. She probably did not think through the process for her choice, but if she had, what might that process be? How can we, as practitioners of health care, apply that same process to assisting our patients and families to cope with the tensions and stresses they encounter? As helping professionals we expect our intervention choices to be based on some sound rationale.

The framework for this process is actually no different from the problem-solving process employed in many other situations and in any other intervention technique: making an assessment through collection of data, identifying the problem, determining the mode of intervention, and then evaluating the results. The difference is that, in this instance, the base is the knowledge and information we have gathered about the concept of humor. We must recognize also that this process has rarely been applied in any systematic way to the use of humor. When humor has been used, more often than not, it has been a spontaneous, intuitive activity rather than a planned one.

It is true that at the present time situational or spontaneous humor is the most common form of humor seen in the health setting. But this may be because humor has not been thought of in any other way. However, by enough conscious, deliberate use of humor, we can make the most out of situational humor which occurs and become skilled enough to begin to be spontaneous and create our own situational humor without always having a preconceived plan. As with any other interpersonal and intervention skill, we integrate the theoretical and problem-solving base into our action, so that the process becomes one that we initiate "almost without thinking." "Practicing" humor has its drawbacks, since if humor seems "practiced" it destroys the humor. However, this is the initial risk we must take if we are ever to become skilled. It is like our first attempts at giving injections or interviewing. We are awkward and hesitant. Yet this is the learning process which is universally accepted.

The first step in the process is assessment, or know your audience! Who is your patient? What is his culture? His age? His personality? What is his sense of humor? What cues can you pick up that he has been using humor as a mechanism for coping? Does he tease and laugh and smile? Does he initiate humor? Make jokes? What are the cues that he would be receptive to your humorous attempts? Have you established the kind of basic relationship of trust and empathy which says to him, "I understand, I'm here to help you. But things aren't so bad. Can't we laugh about it?"

What are the indications that he might not be receptive? Is he emotionally too distraught and too anxious or too angry? Assess his level of anxiety. If it is too high, we know that his decreased ability to concentrate, to listen, to focus may obviate any attempt at humor. Humor might even be irritating or be taken as a negation of his perception of the seriousness of the situation.

We must also assess the patient's physiological condition. Is he in pain? Are drugs clouding his consciousness? Back-stage humor, or humor around the patient but not including him, can be, at this time, irritating and annoying to the patient.

The second step is to determine the problem or the need for which humor might be the choice for intervention. If the patient jokes or uses humor himself, what need is he trying to meet? Evaluate the content of the humor and the situation in which it is occurring. Does it seem to be effective for him in coping with that stress or that need? How have others, including yourself, responded to his humor? Have you encouraged it by laughing and smiling in return and showing your acceptance? Not laughing but responding negatively or with seriousness to a patient's humor should be looked at carefully. Do we insult him or destroy our communication with him because he feels reprimanded?

Once we have made our basic assessment and identified the need or a problem area, we can then determine how, what kind, and when we should initiate the humor, and establish the joke-frame for using it. The humor itself should be based on the professional's own style, the situation, the content and the need, utilizing all the techniques described previously. It may be a witticism, a teasing remark, a joke, or even a funny anecdote that may have happened to another patient in the same circumstance or with the same anxiety.

Once the humorous interaction has occurred, evaluate it. Was it effective? Was the need met? Was the tension reduced? The message conveyed? If so, further intervention may be unnecessary or even inappropriate. One of the functions of humor, as we have repeatedly stated, is to provide a mechanism for dealing with issues and transmitting messages which might be unacceptable if stated directly.

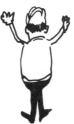

However, rather than getting a laugh, did your humor fall flat? Or did it get a negative response? If it was unsuccessful, analyze why. Was it your technique, was it the humorous content, or was the patient not ready to accept the message? Not many unsuccessful jokes occur, but when they do it may be that "some implicit message not suitable for direct communication is stripped of its camouflage."[4] If the patient responds within a serious frame, failure is implied. It may be that he is reacting to the content of the humor. A slightly risqué joke may be acceptable; a vulgar one may not. Political, racial, or religious jokes may offend. Or somehow the humor failed because the initiator missed some cue or failed to carry out his performance well. It might be helpful to say at that point, to the patient, "Hey, my joke didn't go over very well. I wonder why?"

We might look at two examples of attempts at a practical joke, one of which succeeded and the other failed.

> A patient who had been hospitalized for a long period of time in complete balanced traction was scheduled for further surgery. All of the staff had excellent rapport with the patient. They filled a 5 cc syringe with orange juice, and most of the staff went into the room to help "give" the "preoperative" injection. The staff reported there was a general good feeling by both patient and staff and an evidenced relief of anxiety on the part of the patient.

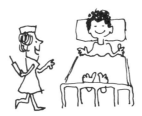

> In another instance, following a hemorrhoidectomy, an enema was ordered for a young male patient; the nurse, who felt she had a good relationship with the patient, thought she would tease him, and brought into the room a huge milk bucket and the largest hose she could find. The patient took one look, ran to the bathroom and refused to come out, unable to see the joke.

In both attempts at humor, the staff felt they had established a good relationship with the patient; yet one failed and the other succeeded. We might wonder if the nurse in the second situation failed to cue the patient that it was a joke! Certainly the pain and embarrassment are more intense with a hemorrhoidectomy than with a preoperative hypodermic, so that the content of the humor was a "touchy" one which the nurse may not have appropriately assessed. There may be other factors contributing to the success or failure which the individuals in the situation could identify if they pursued such an analysis.

Although most humor, as an indirect communication, may serve its purpose without further intervention, humor may also be used as a vehicle for opening up a serious discussion. "A joke may serve as a trial balloon to invite a discussion of doubtful propriety."[5] The negotiations to suspend the general guidelines for joking may be initiated by either party, patient or staff. The health professional and patient may banter back and forth to determine if the other is willing to open a discussion. The more the joker acknowledges that his humor may have a serious import, the easier it is to transpose the humor to a serious discussion. On the other hand, if the patient is not ready to face the taboo topic, he can deny the seriousness and end the negotiation, at which point the staff person should not pursue the topic, but return to the humor facade or terminate the interaction. Such denial indicates to the professional that the patient's use of humor was a face-saving device. In the emotion-laden areas of death and dying the patient or staff "backing off" from joking about dying is very common. On the other hand, humor may also be used as a means for opening up and allowing the patient to discuss his fears and his concerns.

Humor may also be used as a pattern of communication in a long-term relationship to facilitate the therapeutic process. A graduate student in psychiatric nursing working with a young black woman whose acute psychotic episode had been precipitated by her mother's death found that humor became a way of reaching her. The patient's mother had treated her as a retarded child, so that she had felt oppressed and controlled, lacked confidence in herself, was angry at having been thrust in that role. The humorous exchanges and the nurse's use of self-depreciating humor was an attempt to have the patient see her as a friend rather than another controlling mother. For example, when the patient said, she "made spaghetti for dinner last night. It was just canned spaghetti. I'm a can cook," the nurse responded with "You're not alone!" and they both laughed. By the time they were terminating, the patient was calling her "a friend in a professional way" because "a friend knows what you can do."

This same nurse utilized the humor that occurred within a therapy group and picked up on it as a way to integrate the group and relieve tension.

> In one session the patients were talking about how irritating it was when some patients wore soiled clothing and did not bathe. One patient who often used humor, said, "Well, my bath days are Monday and Thursday, but it seems like I never take them on those days. I had one in January..." And as the group started to laugh, the nurse said, "Whether you needed it or not, right, Jack?" At which point another patient quipped, "It was a New Year's resolution!"

The value of the comic effect and humor as a way to control dysfunctional behavior in outer space was suggested early in the space flight programs.[6] The fear, the unknown dangers, the isolation, sensory deprivation, boredom, loss of social contact were some of the sociopsychological stresses identified. Investigators hypothesized that comic laughter could be a means for prevention and amelioration of these reactions. The suggested activities were to provide audiovisual media and tapes of comedy shows, cartoons, classic stories, etc.

However, as the space program progressed, it became evident that the astronauts and staff had incorporated humor into their way of life. Those who followed the space flights and the interchanges between space crew and ground crew heard many quips, little jokes, and humorous comments. When the first ship to reach the moon was taking off to return to the command module, the unexpected strains of *Here We Go into the Wild Blue Yonder* delighted the whole world.

Werner Von Braun in his many talks on "Exploration in Space" used humor to lighten this awesome subject and convey to the audience that it was "just a job." The astronauts often referred to the escape button which detached their compartment during launching in the event of danger as "the chicken switch" and boarding the ship as "walking the plank."

We have referred to the utilization of humor as a technique with individual patients and with groups. We do not mean to neglect the use of humor with families and with children. The same principles and process apply. Humor has been cited as one of the strengthening and coping mechanisms for family living; children and adolescents utilize humor as well in times of illness and respond to humor by staff with the same enthusiasm as adults.

TEACHING HUMOR

Since humor has not been a concept which traditionally has been included in the education of the health professional and there are no present guidelines, how can we begin to teach the practice of humor as a therapeutic tool in the helping process? What learning experiences to utilize humor can we develop for use in the classroom, whether that classroom be part of a basic program, a graduate program, or a continuing education program?

In the chapter on *Humor in Education,* we outlined four areas for the educator to consider. The first two — utilizing humor as a catalyst in the learning process itself, and, facilitating the process of socialization into the health professions — have been discussed. The last two — teaching the concepts and the practice of humor, and modeling the use of humor as a vehicle for facilitating the other three — will be the focus of this section.

The beginning steps for the educator to incorporate humor into the teaching-learning process were outlined in the chapters on *Developing a Sense of Humor* and *The Techniques of Comedy*. Looking at ourselves, assessing our own attitudes and style of humor and then cultivating the basic techniques in creating humor are as vital to our teaching posture as it is to our practice with patients. Modeling the use of humor in the classroom and establishing that kind of relationship provide the vehicle for the student to feel comfortable in relating in this way with patients and colleagues.

In addition to creating personal humor, the teacher, of course, has access to many other humorous articles, cartoons, poems, quotations, posters, and jokes which can be introduced into the class presentation to emphasize a concept or issue or to initiate a discussion. Recently the University of Southern California, in an attempt to lure the students back into the lecture halls, hired a gagwriter to write jokes for professors to use in their lecture courses.*

A small pre-test was conducted of the materials presented in the chapters on *Humor in Education* and *The Techniques of Comedy* on creating humor in the classroom. Twenty-one instructors were asked to read this *Guide for Incorporating Humor in the Teaching-Learning Process,* react to it, and then attempt to use the guide to either add humor to their teaching strategies or to analyze the humor they felt they were already using. They were asked to keep a log for one month, evaluate the usefulness of the *Guide,* and then ask their students to evaluate their performance. The students were not to be told that the study was being conducted until completion.

---

*Time, *Dec 2, 1974.*

Most of the instructors only reacted to the *Guide* and did not test it due to pressures of time or not being involved in enough actual classroom teaching during the period of the study. Several frankly said they had doubts about their ability to do this; others felt the *Guide* was too "cook-bookish" and were uncomfortable with formal jokes. Others, who were already considered "funny" instructors by their peers, suggested that this author review the tapes of their lectures (some of which had been done prior to the study). Twenty of these tapes were subsequently analyzed. Several of the instructors also wrote up material which they had used in their classes. Only two of the group actually tested the *Guide* and had their students evaluate them.

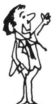

One of these two faculty members honestly felt that she had no sense of humor and was not a "joke-telling" person, but made a deliberate effort to utilize the guidelines. She attempted to be more "light-hearted" and simply "to keep the old Irish maxim, 'you may as well laugh grief as cry it.'" She made more frequent attempts to laugh over minor errors and felt, thus, she was less threatening to the students. She utilized a slide-cartoon series called *The Long Ranger* in a class on Perspective Medicine, discussing long-range planning for health care and health hazard appraisal. The series is a take-off on the Lone Ranger; she introduced the audiovisual aid with a comment that this was to be enjoyed and students should not try to take notes.

Interestingly enough the students' evaluations of her ranged from not noticing any change to yes, there was one. One student noticed the instructor was "very cheerful, but thought it was spring fever!" Moreover, despite the instructor's perception of herself as "not humorous," two of the students felt there was nothing unusual because this instructor was always in good humor, ready to tell a joke or laugh at another joke or funny situation, and didn't see how she could become more humorous "without being ridiculous."

The other instructor who utilized the Guide and had her students evaluate her was one whom everyone felt was absolutely the funniest instructor around. Yet the instructor said, "They laugh, but I don't know why they do." In this instance, she asked another instructor to observe her in class and record those instances in which laughter occurred. In addition, this author reviewed the tapes of her lectures. The analysis showed that her humor consisted primarily of very spontaneous, situational witticisms which came out in such a dry, droll fashion that the delivery was as important to the humorous communication as the content itself. The content is typical of situational humor that taken out of context may not be funny at all. One needs to be involved in the situation to get the full impact of the amusement. One student commented that the instructor had a mischievous twinkle in her eye that suggested "chronic humor." Are these cues to the attitude about which we have been talking?

She very often mispronounced words, like "eveel" for evil and "royal" for rural and then added as the students laughed, "I hear you! I should take a course in diction."

Other examples:

> When the class asked her "to slow down" in her lecturing, she responded with "...slow down? Sorry, I did say we'd mosey on through the respiratory unit, didn't I?"

> In attempting to draw on the blackboard a sketch of the pedicle of the kidney, with which she was having difficulty, she said, "I can't wait till we get to kidneys. I can draw those!"

In describing how to count seconds, she said one should say to oneself, "...1001, 1002, 1003.... Is that right?"

In talking about loss of time sense in a particular disease, she said "Time sure flies when you're having fun."

She used herself in many situations, *e.g.,* describing her own habit of smoking when talking about emphysema.

Fifty-six of her 100 students evaluated her; again, the comments ranged from very positive statements about her humor to one who did not notice anything funny! This verifies the fact that humor is a matter of individual perception and receptivity.

The students were asked if the humor improved the class and increased learning. The responses were generally positive. It made the class "less dull," "provided a relaxed atmosphere more conducive to learning," and made the instructor "seem more human." "One seems to remember facts when they are associated with something funny and interesting." Humor "revives lagging attention." "Kept me awake." "Alleviated the anxiety associated with learning."

An analysis of the humor from the 20 tapes plus the written descriptions of humor used could be broken down into three major categories:

1. spontaneous, situational humor;
2. canned variety;
3. reference to humor or use of humor;

and two sub-categories, those that:

1. related to the topic or subject of the lecture.
2. were extraneous to the subject matter.

In listening to the lecture there were many times that laughter occurred which must have related to a gesture, facial expression, or some other nonverbal cues which the listener could not see and, therefore, could not evaluate the reason for the laughter.

The amount of data collected was too small to be statistically analyzed in any significant way. Most of the incidents of humor were of the spontaneous situational type. Many of them were simple pleasantries. They were about equally divided between those directly related to the subject and those external to the topic. A directly related example of humor occurred during a panel discussion on kidney transplants.

> One of the students asked if patients who needed transplants wait anxiously for donors. One of the head nurses on the panel responded. "I asked my patients if they lay awake on Memorial Day weekend listening for screeching brakes and they only laughed. Of course there is a shortage of donors since the speed limit was set at 55!"

Humor external to the subject area was an aside: "Is it hot in here or am I going through menopause?" And then followed some quips about age and *Premarin* ads.

Humor of the canned variety consisted of those already prepared jokes, cartoons, poems, etc. During a class on obesity, the instructor used several of these. She gave some definitions of fad diets: "A rhythm method to girth control" or "A grim cycle of lose-a-little, gain a little more." She opened the class with this poem on a transparency.

> Fading is the taper waist,
> Shapeless grows the shapely limb,
> And although severely laced,
> Spreading is the figure trim,
> Stouter than I used to be,
> Still more corpulent grow I.
> There will be too much of me
> In the coming bye and bye.
>
> *Gilbert and Sullivan*

There were two references to humor itself. The "funny" instructor several times said, "Write all those jokes down, I'll use them again next year." Another instructor in discussing crisis intervention was relating her own crisis when her gynecologist during an examination asked, "When did you notice the lump in your breast?" She said to the class, "I responded by making a joke.

That's my coping mechanism. But he didn't laugh, which said to me, it is serious. Instead he asked if I had a choice of a surgeon."

This study is only a beginning in analyzing humor in the classroom and evaluating methods for learning to model it. The feedback regarding the guidelines themselves were helpful. The one major accomplishment of the study was the change in attitude regarding the cultivation of humor expressed by many of the educators. As one educator said, who initially admitted to feeling dubious about such a *Guide* based on "you either had it or didn't..."

> Consciously thinking about humor is the first step rather than envying the person who is "naturally witty." I suppose we all have self-conscious fears of coming across poorly and using humor alien to our style. Yet there is only one way to find out what one is comfortable with and can use effectively.

The other aspect an educator must consider is how to teach the intervention skills to her students. What kind of learning experiences can we provide once the basic theoretical content is given? There are several suggested methods which could be used.

To help students to look at their own styles and attitudes toward humor, they could be asked to write down or relate either a favorite joke or the funniest thing that ever happened to them. An analysis of the joke is also a way to evaluate their knowledge of the basic concept. This might be done as an individual assignment or a group activity.

Role-playing situations in the classroom in which humor is used might be another learning activity. This can be a demonstration by the instructor or an assignment to the students. Brief descriptions of patient situations in which some basic feeling such as tension, anxiety, anger, or embarrassment is evident can be developed. Utilizing these, the students make an assessment and then role-play how they would relieve these feelings through humor. In management classes, at graduate and continuing education levels, how staff might approach management about problems and issues, or how administrators might approach staff in supervising, evaluating or making changes through the avenue of humor can be role-played. Any of these may be a spontaneous classroom activity or an overnight assignment so that the student deliberately plans an intervention. Role-playing in the classroom helps to relieve anxiety and makes the anticipated situation in reality less awkward.

In a beginning class in nursing, two instructors demonstrated how humor can be used to reduce a patient's anxiety during preoperative care. First, the instructors played the role in a very negative way, with loud and raucous joking remarks to each other, asking the patient if she wanted her gallstones in a bottle so she could display them on her mantel at home. The "patient" obviously cringed and grimaced and huddled under the sheets. Then the scene was replayed in a positive fashion, using a joke to initiate a conversation about her fears. The "nurse" said, "You look as though you'd like to get out of bed and run. You remind me of a cartoon I saw. There is an operating room with six gowned and masked figures standing around an empty operating room table. The surgeon is looking around and saying 'Come, come, now, *one* of you must be the patient.'" The role-playing "patient" giggled and said, "Yeah, that's what I'd like to do, hide!" A discussion of her fears ensued.

The faculty role-playing or demonstrating some skill in a very negative way often is very humorous because of its absurdity and gets lots of laughs. This can be a means for saying, "All right, how would you do this appropriately?"

The instructor also being able to relate her own humorous experiences as a student or staff nurse helps the student, who usually has unrealistic expectations for herself, to relax and feel that she can laugh at her own mistakes if the teacher can laugh at hers. Making use of situation humor in the classroom also adds to the instructor's humanness. On one occasion the instructor, who was demonstrating how to move a patient in bed, first took her shoes off (high heels), next her glasses which had fallen down, and then remarked, "I promise you, that's the last thing I'll take off."

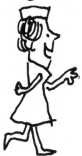

There may be a variety of other learning experiences which could be devised for "practicing" the use of humor. Of course, encouraging the student to add humor to her assessment of patients in planning nursing care in the clinical area provides the opportunity for the actual experience necessary to develop the skill in intervention.

SUMMARY

There are still many unanswered questions in this whole area of humor and much more research to be done. But, we need to begin. We need to explore the use of this tool, to try out various approaches, to experiment.

The DK theory is what we operate on in most helping relationships, anyway, says one authority. DK stands for degrees of knowledge, ranging from *don't know* to *damn konfident!*

The DK theory is very simply applied: To each and every professional action, the worker simply attaches a mental subscript, DK = ____%, referring to the percentage or proportion of ignorance actually operating in this particular action. One must act on the best available knowledge, to be sure, but one must be equally aware of the degree of knowledge involved in one's actions.[7]

So, let us have the courage to try. After all, jokes never really "killed" anyone!

REFERENCES

1. Emerson JP, *Social Functions of Humor*, p 47-48.
2. Fry WF Jr, *Sweet Madness*, p 161.
3. Handelman D, Kapferer B: Forms of joking activity: a comparative approach. *Am Anthropologist* 74:484-517, 1972.
4. Emerson, *Social Functions of Humor*, p 150.
5. Emerson JP: Negotiating the serious import of humor. *Sociometry* 32:169-81, 1969, p 172.
6. Friedman LA: Use of comic effect for control of dysfunctional human behavior in outer space. *Human Factors*, pp 355-358, August 1963.
7. Bloom M: *The Paradox of Helping. Introduction to the Philosophy of Scientific Practice*. New York, John Wiley and Sons, Inc, 1975, p 82.

BIBLIOGRAPHY

Powell BS: Laughter and healing: the uses of humor in hospitals treating children. *Association for the Care of Children in Hospitals Journal*, pp 10-16, November, 1974.

Wessell ML Sister: Use of humor by an immobilized adolescent girl during hospitalization. *Maternal Child Nursing Journal*, pp 35-48, Spring 1975.

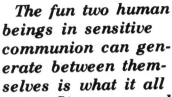

The fun two human beings in sensitive communion can generate between themselves is what it all comes down to. We make ourselves happy by making each other happy. And why not? We are all so capable of making each other miserable that the telling of jokes, or the communication of humor in general seems an indispensable balance in the seesaw of human relations.[2]

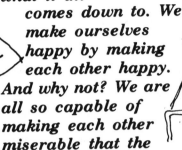

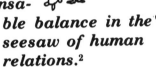

conclusions

Harvey Mindess has said it so well. Laughter is indispensable. We must learn how to develop it, to cultivate it, to use it in a more forceful way. The purpose of this book has been to pull together the available knowledge in the area of humor as a beginning in this effort. We have only scratched the surface. There is much more to be done.

The initial studies attempted for the development of this book were exploratory in nature. What has been revealed are the areas needed for further research.

1. First and foremost, more definitive reliable methods

and tools for studying humor and for the collection of humorous data in natural settings are needed. The difficulties encountered by this author have been a problem to others: the need to be a direct observer of the humor, yet the paradox of getting "caught up in the humor" and forgetting to record or be objective; influencing the reduction or increase in humor by the presence of a "collector of humor"; the long periods of time necessary to collect enough data for meaningful results; the unreliability of data reported by others because of individual perceptions and receptivity; and the difficulty in categorizing the data collected.

2. Current descriptions of humor in all of the natural settings in the area of health and illness are needed. Those which have been done are hospital-related and were completed in the late Fifties and early Sixties.

3. More specifically, within this description of humor in the health setting, research on what makes the humor successful and what factors destroy it or cause the attempt to fail is needed.

4. Definitive studies of the use of humor related to culture or ethnic groups is needed, specifically related to its use in health and illness.

5. Studies on the use of humor in current community mental health settings and in relation to current humanistic psychotherapies are needed since psychoanalytic theory has dominated past research.

6. There is a need for developmental theories of humor and humor related to all the age groups.

7. Research in the area of humor and learning theory must be done, as well as research in the methodologies for teaching humor.

8. And lastly, research in the whole untried and pioneer area of intervention is of prime importance and is the ultimate goal of the study of humor.

In conclusion, in my enthusiasm and strong belief in the value of humor, I may have projected a one-sided view: that humor is all! Perhaps you have already recognized for yourself and accepted that, because humor has been so neglected, I have been rather adamant. However, I feel impelled to remind the health professional that humor must always be placed in perspective to the whole, that whole a human being called *MAN*.

In the total plan for the care of our patient, humor is *one* communication tool, *one* mechanism for coping, *one* teaching methodology. It is useful and therapeutic in the right situation and the right time. As with anything else, a good thing can be overdone; a judicious amount is the right amount. If a drug is good, three times the dosage is not better. There will be times, as with grief when there is a need for lightness and humor, that humor will turn to tears, when laughter no longer suffices. What is important is to understand humor, to become skilled in recognizing when it is appropriate and beneficial, and to encourage, not ignore, it.

In this age of rapid medical and technological advances, when the fears and threats of being replaced and controlled by machines are a reality, humor can be the means for retaining the humanness in the health professions. Humor is exclusively a human condition. Adlai Stevenson once paraphrased Socrates' famous statement, "The unexamined life is not worth living," with "Life without laughter is not worth examining."

REFERENCES

1. Mindess, *Laugher and Liberation,* p 172.

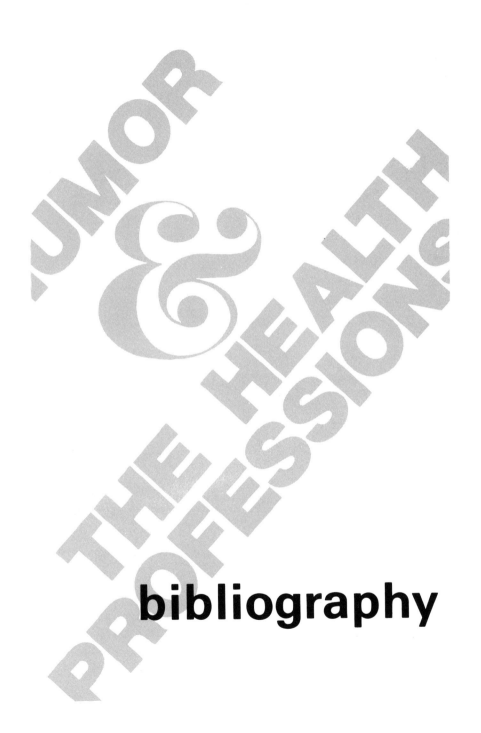

bibliography

bibliography

Adair, John; Deuschle, Kurt W: *The People's Health, Medicine and Anthropology in a Navajo Community.* New York: Appleton-Century-Crofts, 1970.

Adams, Joey: *Encyclopedia of Humor.* New York: The Bobbs-Merrill Company, Inc., 1968.

Adams, Wesley J: The use of sexual humor in teaching human sexuality at the university level. *Family Coordinator* (October 1974), 365-368.

Allport, Gordon W: *The Individual and His Religion.* New York: The Macmillan Company, 1961.

Andrew, Richard J: The origin of facial expression. *Scientific American* (October 1965), 88-94.

Armour, Richard: *The Medical Muse.* New York: McGraw Hill Book Company, 1963.
: A short course in geriatric medicine. *Geriatrics* (Jan 1974), 125-129.

Baker, Robert A: *Psychology in the Wry.* Princeton, N.J.: D. Van Nostrand Company, 1963.
: *A Stress Analysis of a Strapless Evening Gown and Other Essays for a Scientific Age.* Englewood Cliffs, N.J.: Prentice-Hall, Inc., 1967.

Bergson, Henri. Laughter. [1900] *In* Enck, John J.; Forter, Elizabeth T.; and Whitley, Alvin (eds). *The Comic in Theory and Practice.* New York: Appleton-Century-Crofts, 1960, pp 43-64.

Bergler, Edmund: *Laughter and the Sense of Humor.* New York: Intercontinental Medical Book Corp., 1956.

Berkowitz Leonard: Aggressive humor as a stimulus to aggressive responses. *Journal of Personality and Social Psychology* 16:710-717 (Apr) 1970.

Berlyne, D.E.: Laughter, humor and play. *Handbook of Social Psychology* 3:795-813, 1969.

Bloom, Martin: *The Paradox of Helping:* Introduction to the Philosophy of Scientific Practice. New York: John Wiley and Sons, 1975.

Bornemeier, W.C.: Sphincter-Protecting Hemorrhoidectomy. *American Journal of Proctocology* 11:48-52, 1960.

Bowen, Elenore Smith [pseud]: *Return to Laughter.* Garden City, N.Y.: The Natural History Library, Anchor Books, Doubleday and Company, 1964.

Bradney, Pamela: The joking relationship in industry. *Human Relations* 14:170-187, 1957.

Brody, Morris W.: The meaning of laughter. *Psychoanalytic Quarterly* 19:192-201, 1950.

Brown, Jo: *Perennially Yours, PROBIE.* New York: Springer Publishing Company, 1958.

Burma, John H.: Humor as a technique in race conflict. *American Sociological Review* 11:710-715, 1946.

Byrne, Don: The relationship between humor and the expression of hostility. *Journal of Abnormal and Social Psychology* 53:84-89, 1955.

Coser, Rose Laub: Some social functions of laughter. *Human Relations* 12:171-182, 1959.

——: Laughter among colleagues. *Psychiatry* 23:81-95, 1960.

——: Some social functions of laughter. *In* Ed. Skipper, James K. Jr.; and Leonard, Robert C. (eds): *Social Interaction and Patient Care.* Philadelphia: J.B. Lippincott, 1965, pp 292-306.

Deloria, Vine Jr: Indian humor. *Custer Died for Your Sins.* New York: Macmillan Co., 1969.

Dobree, Bonamy: Restoration comedy, drama and values. *In* Felheim, Marvin (ed): *Comedy: Plays, Theory and Criticism.* New York: Harcourt, Brace and World, 1962, pp 202-205.

Dunn, H.L.: High level wellness for man and society. *American Journal of Public Health* 49:786-792, 1959.

Eastman, M.: *The Sense of Humor.* New York: Scribners, 1921.

——: *The Enjoyment of Laughter.* New York: Simon and Schuster, 1936.

Eble, Kenneth: *A Perfect Education.* New York: Macmillan Company, 1966.

Emerson, Joan Paret: Social functions of humor in a hospital setting. Ph.D. dissertation, University of California, 1963.

——: Negotiating the serious import of humor. *Sociometry* 32:169-181, 1969.

Enck, John J.; Forter, Elizabeth T.; Whitley, Alvin, (eds.): *The Comic in Theory and Practice.* New York: Appleton-Century-Crofts, 1960.

Engel, George: *Psychological Development in Health and Disease.* Philadelphia: W.B. Saunders, 1962.

Eysenck, H.J.: An experimental analysis of five tests of appreciation of humor. *Educational and Psychological Measurement* 3:191-214, 1943.

——: Foreword. Goldstein, Jeffrey H.; and McGhee, Paul E. (eds): *The Psychology of Humor.* New York: Academic Press, 1972, pp xiii-xvii.

Eysenck, H.J.; Eysenck, S.B.G.: *Eysenck Personality Inventory.* San Diego: Educational and Industrial Testing Service, 1963.

Felheim, Marvin: *Comedy: Plays, Theory, and Criticism.* New York: Harcourt, Brace and World, 1962.

Flugel, J.C.: Humor and laughter. *In* Lindsay, Gardner (ed): *Handbook of Social Psychology.* Cambridge, Mass.: Addison-Wesley, 1954, pp 709-734.

Fox, Renee C.: *Experiment Perilous.* Glencoe, Ill.: The Free Press, A. Corporation, 1959.

Fox, Renee C.; Swazey, Judith P. *The Courage to Fail:* A Social View of Organ Transplants and Dialysis. Chicago: The University of Chicago Press, 1974.

Foster, Herbert L.: *Ribbin', Jivin', and Playin' the Dozens. The Unrecognized Dilemma of Inner City Schools.* Cambridge, Mass.: Ballinger Publishing Company, 1974.

Frankl, Viktor: *Man's Search for Meaning.* New York: Washington Square Press, 1963.

Freud, Sigmund: *Jokes and Their Relation to the Unconscious.* [1905]. *In* Strachey,

James (ed): *The Complete Psychological Works of Sigmund Freud,* vol VIII. London: Hogarth Press, 1961.

: Humor. *In* Strachey, James (ed): *The Complete Psychological Works of Sigmund Freud,* (1923). London: Hogarth Press, 1961.

Friedman, Lee A.: Use of comic effect for control of dysfunctional human behavior in outer space. *Human Factors* 5:355-362, 1963.

Frost, Robert: Forgive, O Lord. *In the Clearing.* New York: Holt, Rinehart and Winston, 1962.

Fry, William F., Jr.: *Sweet Madness:* A Study of Humor. Palo Alto, Ca.: Pacific Books, Publishers, 1963.

Goldstein, Jeffrey H.; McGhee, Paul E.: *The Psychology of Humor.* Theoretical Perspectives and Empirical Issues. New York: Academic Press, 1972.

Goodrich, Anne T.; Jules, Henry; Goodrich, D. Walls: Laughter in psychiatric staff conferences: a sociopsychiatric analysis. *American Journal of Orthopsychiatry* 24:175-184, 1954.

Grotjahn, Martin: *Beyond Laughter.* New York: The Blakiston Division, McGraw Hill Company, 1957.

: Sexuality and humor — don't laugh. *Psychology Today* July:51-53, 1972.

Gutman, Jonathan; Priest, Robert F.: When is aggression funny? *Journal of Personality and Social Psychology* 12(1):60-65, 1969.

Harms, Ernest: The development of humor. *Journal of Abnormal and Social Psychology* 38:351-369, 1943.

Handelman, Don; Kapferer, Bruce: Forms of joking activity: a comparative approach. *American Anthropologist* 74:484-517, 1972.

Harrel, Stewart: *When It's Laughter You're After.* Norman, Okla.: University of Oklahoma Press, 1962.

Hayworth, D.: The social origins and functions of laughter. *Psychological Review* 35:367-384, 1928.

Hazlitt, William: Lecture on "Wit and Humor" (1819). *In* Enck, John J.; Forter, Elizabeth T.; and Whitley, Alvin (eds): *The Comic In Theory and Practice.* New York: Appleton-Century-Crofts, 1960, pp 16-21.

Heller, Joseph: *Catch 22.* New York: Dell Publishing Company, 1955.

Hill, Hamlin: Black humor: its cause and cure. *Colorado Quarterly* XVII:57-64, 1968.

Hill, Willard: *Navajo Humor.* Menasha: Banta, 1943.

Hines, Ralph H.: Health status of black Americans. *In* Jaco, Gantley E (ed): *Patients, Physicians and Illness,* 2nd ed. New York: The Free Press, 1972. pp 40-50.

Jahoda, Marie: *Current Concepts of Positive Mental Health.* New York: Basic Books, 1958.

Kaplan, Howard; Boyd, Ina H.: The social functions of humor on an open psychiatric ward. *Psychiatric Quarterly* 39:502-515, 1965.

Kelley, Earl C.: The fully functioning self. *Perceiving Behaving Becoming:* A New Focus for Education. Washington, D.C.: Association for Supervision and Curriculum Development, National Education Association, Yearbook, 1962.

Kesey, Ken: *One Flew Over the Cuckoo's Nest.* New York: Signet Books, 1962.

Kevin, Sister Mary: How to recognize your patient's "humors." *RN* Dec:51-53, 1964.

Klapp, O.: The fool as a social type. *American Journal of Sociology* 55:157-162, 1950.

Kluckhohn, Clyde; Leighton, Dorothea Cross: *The Navajo.* Cambridge: Harvard University Press, 1946.

Koestler, Arthur: *The Act of Creation.* New York: The Macmillan Company, 1964.

Krill, Donald F.: Existential psychotherapy and the problem of anomie. *Social Work* April:33-49, 1969.

Kronenberger, Louis. *The Thread of Laughter.* New York: Alfred A. Knopf, 1952.

Kubie, Lawrence S. The destructive potential of humor in psychotherapy. *American Journal of Psychiatry,* 127 (January 1971), 861-866.

Landon, Melville D. *Wit and Humor of the Age.* Chicago: Star Publishing Company, 1883.

Lefrancois, Guy R. *Psychological Theories and Human Learning: Kongor's Report.* Monterey, Calif.: Brooks-Cole Publishing Company, 1972.

Leighton, Alexander and Leighton, Dorothea Cross. *The Navajo Door.* Cambridge: Harvard Press, 1944.

Leininger, Madeleine. *Nursing and Anthropology: Two Worlds to Blend.* New York: John Wiley and Sons, Inc., 1970.

Levine, Jacob. Responses to humor. *Scientific American,* 194, No. 2)2 (February 1956), 31-35.

_____. Regression in primitive clowning. *Psychoanalytic Quarterly,* 30 (1961), 72-83.

_____. Humor. *International Encyclopedia of the Social Sciences.* Ed. David Sills. New York: The Macmillan Company, 1968. VII, 1-7.

Levine, Jacob and Redlich, Frederick. Failure to understand humor. *Psychoanalytic Quarterly,* 24 (1955), 560-572.

Lorenz, Konrad. *On Aggression.* New York: Harcourt, Brace and World, Inc., 1963.

Lundy, David and Mettee, David. Evaluation of an aggressor as a function of exposure to cartoon humor. *Journal of Personality and Social Psychology,* 12(1):66-71, 1969.

Madsen, William: *The Mexican-Americans of South Texas.* New York: Holt, Rinehart and Winston, 1964.

Maslow, A.H.: *Motivation and Personality,* 2nd ed. New York: Harper and Row, 1970.

McCabe, Gracia S.: Cultural influences on patient behavior. *The American Journal of Nursing* 60(8):1101-1104, 1960.

McDougall, William: An instinct of laughter. *An Introduction to Social Psychology.* New York: University Paperbacks, Barnes and Noble, 1963.

McGhee, Paul E.: Development of the humor response: a review of the literature. *Psychological Bulletin* 76:328-348, 1971.

McLuhan, Marshall: *The Medium is the Massage.* New York: Bantam Books, 1967.

Mendel, Werner (ed.): *A Celebration of Laughter.* Los Angeles: Mara Books, 1970.

Meredith, George: On comedy and the uses of the comic spirit. Lecture, 1877. *In* Felheim, Marvin (ed): *Comedy: Plays, Theory, and Criticism.* New York: Harcourt, Brace and World, Inc., 1962, pp 205-214.

Middleton, Russell; Moland, John: Humor in Negro and White subcultures: a study of jokes among university students. *American Sociological Review* 24:61-69, 1959.

Mikes, GEORGE: *Laughing Matter.* New York: The Library Press, 1971.

Mindess, Harvey: *Laughter and Liberation.* Los Angeles: Nash Publishing Company, 1971.

Monro, D.H.: *Argument of Laughter.* Melbourne: Melbourne University Press, 1951.

Mosak, Harold H.; Dreikurs, Rudolf: Adlerian psychotherapy. *In* Corsini, Raymond (ed): *Current Psychotherapies.* Itasca, Ill.: F.E. Peacock Publishers, 1973, pp 35-83.

Murphy, Brian; Pollio, Howard R.: I'll laugh if you will. *Psychology Today* Dec:106-109, 1973.

Myrdal, G.: *An American Dilemma.* New York: Harper, 1944.

Nava, Julian: Foreword. *In* Wagner, Nathaniel N.; Haug, Marsha J. (eds): *Chicanos: Social and Psychological Perspectives.* Saint Louis: C.V. Mosby Company, 1971, pp xxi-xxiii.

Norris, Catherine: Greetings from a lonely crowd. *Nursing Forum* 1:73-82, 1961-62.

Nussbaum, K.; Michaux, W.W.: Response to humor in depression: a predictor and evaluator of patient change. *Psychiatric Quarterly* 37:527-539, 1963.

Obrdlik, Antonio J.: Gallows humor — a sociological phenomenon. *American Journal of Sociology* 47:709-716, 1942.

O'Connell, Walter E.: The adaptive functions of wit and humor. *Journal of Abnormal and Social Psychology* 61(2):263-270, 1960.

　: An item analysis of the wit and humor appreciation test. *The Journal of Social Psychology* 50:271-276, 1962.

　: Multidimensional investigation of Freudian humor. *Psychiatry Quarterly* 38:97-108, 1964.

　: Resignation, humor and wit. *Psychoanalytic Review* 51:49-56, 1964.

　: Humor and death. *Psychological Reports* 22:391-402, 1968.

　: Creativity in humor. *The Journal of Social Psychology* 78:237-241, 1969.

　: The social aspects of wit and humor. *The Journal of Social Psychology* 79:183-187, 1969.

　: Peterson, Penny: Humor and repression. *Journal of Existential Psychiatry*, 4:309-316, 1964.

　: Covert, Charles: Death attitudes and humor appreciation among medical students. *Existential Psychiatry* 6:433-442, 1967.

　　Rothhaus, Paul; Hanson, Philip G.; Moyer, Ray: Jest appreciation and interaction in leaderless groups. *International Journal of Group Psychotherapy* 19:454-462, 1969.

Olendzki, Margaret: *Cautionary Tales.* Wakefield, Mass.: Contemporary Publishing Company, 1973.

Orben, Robert: The Pied Piper of humor. *Talent.* Cleveland, Ohio: International Platform Association, Spring, 1972, pp 34-36.

Pape, Jane: *Psimplified Psychiatry.* New Jersey: Stuart James Publishing Company, 1968.

Parsons, Talcott: Definitions of health and illness in light of American values and social structure. *In* Jaco E.C. (ed): *Patients, Physicians and Illness.* New York: The Free Press, 1958.

Pearson, Gayle Angus: A child's humor. *Nursing Science* 3:95-108, 1965.

Piddington, Ralph: *The Psychology of Laughter.* New York: Gamut Press, 1933, 1963.

Poland, Warren S.: The place of humor in psychotherapy. *American Journal of Psychiatry* 128:635-637, 1971.

Powell, Barbara S.: Laughter and healing: the use of humor in hospitals treating children. *Association for the Care of Children in Hospitals Journal,* Nov:10-16, 1974.

Radcliffe-Brown, A.R.: On joking relationships. *Africa* 13:195-210, 1940.

　: On joking relationships. *Structure and Function in Primitive Society.* New York: The Free Press, 1952.

Rapp, A.: *The Origins of Wit and Humor.* New York: Dutton, 1951.

Redlich, Frederick C.; Levine, Jacob; Sohler, Theodore P.: A mirth response test: preliminary report on a psycho-diagnostic technique utilizing dynamics of humor. *American Journal of Orthopsychiatry* 21:717-734, 1951.

Reese, R.L.: Does humor have a place in scientific writing? *American Medical Writers' Association Bulletin* 17:11-13, 1967.

Reichard, Gladys: *Navajo Religion, A Study of Symbolism.* New York: Bolligen Foundation, 1950.

Robinson, Vera M.: Humor in nursing. *In* Carlson, Carolyn E. (coordinator): *Behavioral Concepts and Nursing Intervention.* Philadelphia: J.B. Lippincott, 1970, pp 129-150.

Rogers, Carl: *Freedom to Learn.* Columbus, Ohio: Charles E. Merrill, 1969.

Rogers, E.S.: *Human Ecology and Health.* New York: The Macmillian Company, 1960.

Roland, Charles G.: Thoughts about medical writing: can it be funny and medical? *Anesthesia and Analgesia... Current Researches,* 50(2):Mar-Apr, 1971.

Rose, Gilbert J.: King Lear and the use of humor in treatment. *Journal of the American Psychoanalytic Association* 12:927-940, 1969.

Sanders, Donald H.: *Computers in Society.* New York: McGraw Hill, 1973.

Schoel, Doris R.; Busse, Thomas V.: Humor and creative abilities. *Psychological Reports* 29:34, 1971.

Schulz, Max F.: *Black Humor Fiction in the Sixties.* Athens, Ohio: Ohio University Press, 1973.

Simmons, Donald: Protest humor: folkloristic reaction to prejudice. *American Journal of Psychiatry,* 120:567-570, 1963.

Singer, David L.; Berkowitz, Leonard: Differing creativities in the wit and the clown. *Perceptual and Motor Skills* 35:3-6, 1972.

Smith, Ewart E.; White, Helen L.: Wit, creativity and sarcasm. *Journal of Applied Psychology* 49:131-134, 1965.

Spitz, Rene: The smiling response: a contribution to the ontogenesis of social relations. *Genetic Psychology Monographs* 34:57-125, 1946.

Steiner, Stan: *The New Indians.* New York: Harper and Row, 1968.

Stephenson, R.M.: Conflict and control functions of humor. *American Journal of Sociology* 56:569-574, 1959.

Stuart, I.R.: Primary and secondary process as reflections of catastrophe: the political cartoon as an instrument of group emotional dynamics. *Journal of Social Psychology,* Dec:231-239, 1964.

Sully, James: Essay on laughter, 1902. *The Psychology of Laughter: A Study in Social Adaptation.* 1933 reissued; New York: Gamut Press, 1963, pp 196-200.

Thompson, Seth: The trickster cycle. *The Folktale.* New York: The Dryden Press, 1946, pp 319-328.

Vargas, Manuel J.: Uses of humor in group psychotherapy. *Group Psychotherapy* 14:198-202, 1961.

Wessell, Sister Mary Louise: Use of humor by an immobilized adolescent girl during hospitalization. *Maternal-Child Nursing Journal* 4(1):35-48, 1975.

White, E.S.: Some remarks on humor. *The Second Tree from the Corner.* New York: Harper and Brothers, 1954. *In* Enck, John J.; Forter, Elizabeth T.; and Whitley, Alvin (eds): *The Comic in Theory and Practice.* New York: Appleton-Century-Crofts, 1960, pp 102-108.

Whiting, Percy: *How to Speak and Write with Humor.* New York: McGraw Hill Company, 1969.

Wolfenstein, Martha: *Children's Humor.* Glencoe, Ill.: Free Press, 1954.

Zwerling, Israel: The favorite joke in diagnostic and therapeutic interviewing. *Psychoanalytic Quarterly* 24:104-114, 1955.

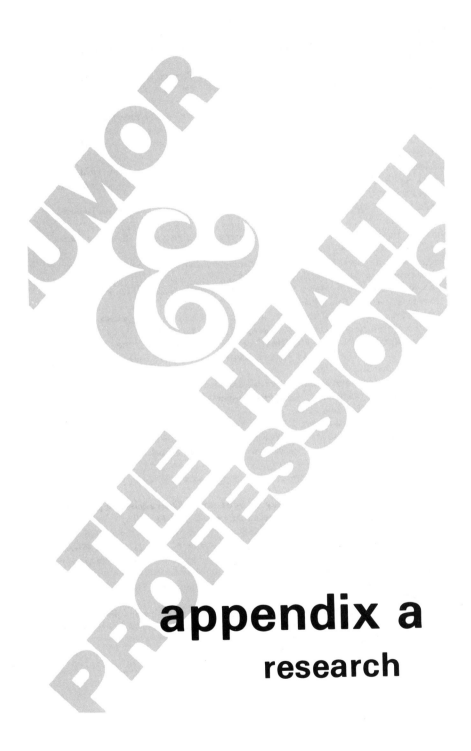

appendix a
research

research

A Study of Humorous Interactions in Health Settings Involving Patients from Three Specific Cultures: Black-American, Spanish-American, and American Indian

I. Introduction

There have been several studies attempting to determine the nature of humor used in health settings (Coser, 1959; Fox, 1959; Emerson, 1964; Robinson, 1970; Meechan, 1973). The humor has been found to be an indirect form of communication, subordinated to the formal patterns of communication. Humor as a coping mechanism can be initiated either by the patient or the professional for a variety of purposes such as: to decrease social distance; to establish relationships; to relieve anxiety, stress, or tension; to release anger or frustration; to avoid or deny feelings; or to facilitate the expression of feelings.

Much humor that occurs, however, is spontaneous and unplanned. Despite our recognition of its value and beliefs, we have not attempted to analyze or understand it in order to make conscious, deliberate use of humor as a tool in communication during professional interventions. It is the contention of this investigator that humor is constructive and healthy and its use as a coping mechanism should be encouraged; that humor can be understood and cultivated and learned by the professional.

In the planned use of humor in interactions, however, there are many variables to be considered. One of these is the cultural background of the patient. Does culture or ethnicity make a difference in the kind of humor which is appreciated? Is there a relationship between a specific culture and its use of humor in times of stress such as illness? If so, what is it? Would the culture of the patient make a difference in the professional's use of humor if the professional were a nonmember of that culture?

A review of the literature of three cultures — Black-American, Spanish-American, and American Indian — reveals a lack of study and research in ıship to these questions around the use of humor by specific cultures ıtresses of illness. There is a need to collect some original data and to describe the use of humor in health situations in which the patient is from another culture.

II. Statement of the Problem

The focus of this study will be to investigate humorous interactions between patients from one of the three cultures and the professionals caring for them during the professional-client relationship.

III. Statement of the Purpose

It is the purpose of this exploratory study to observe, describe, and develop a beginning knowledge of the use of humor by patients from another culture in the health situation by:
1. Identifying those situations in which humor occurs between patient and professional, the patient being from the Black-American, Spanish-American, or American Indian culture, and initiated either by the patient or the professional.
2. Identifying whether humor is a pattern of communication by the persons of the three cultures in times of health-illness situations.
3. Identifying the cultural differences, if they exist, in the humor used in these situations.
4. Identifying the differences in the humorous interaction when
   a. the professional is an Anglo.
   b. the professional is a member of the same culture.
   c. the professional is a member of one of the other two cultures.
5. Collecting and analyzing the data in relationship to the problems stated.
6. Organizing the results of this study into a body of knowledge which can be used by the professional in his planned use of humor in professional-patient interactions.

IV. Definition of Terms

Humorous interactions: No single definition of humor has been acceptable to all investigators in this area. Much time has been spent attempting to differentiate between the various forms of humor such as wit, satire, comedy, jokes, etc. Humor has been considered to be present when there is some behavioral manifestation such as laughter or smiling, which are the standard responses. However, the response can be also a change in facial expression or tone of voice, twinkling eyes, or other indications of amusement.

In this study humor is viewed in a social context as a medium of communication. Therefore, for the purpose of this study, humor will be defined, in a more comprehensive sense, as any communication which is perceived by any of the interacting parties as humorous and leads to laughing, smiling, or feeling of amusement. This might include teasing, jocular talk, witticisms, puns, and clowning as well as joke-telling or a practical joke.

Health setting: The health setting is defined as a situation or place in which a health professional is caring for or interacting with a patient. This includes hospital ward, emergency room, clinic, neighborhood health center, office, home, etc.

Health professional: The term *health professional* is used broadly to encompass any member of the health team and is used simply to make a distinction between patient and health care giver.

V. Methodology

Basic study design: The basic design employed will be a non-experimental descriptive survey. The descriptive approach was chosen because of the fact that data concerning the use of humor in times of illness by persons from the three cultures are nonexistent. The goal of the descriptive method is to obtain meaningful information pertaining to the phenomenon under study in order to discover new facts which can later be tested. The nonexperimental approach was selected because the study necessitated observation in the original setting without control over environmental factors.

Sample: Two large general hospitals, a public health agency, and several clinics and neighborhood health centers in areas where a large number of persons from the three cultures reside will be asked to participate. Selected nurses employed in these settings as well as other members of the health team who are willing to cooperate will be asked to record humorous interactions with patients from any of the three cultures. These interactions may be ones in which they participated or those in which they observed other professionals interacting with patients. Health professionals from the three cultures will be used, as well as white or Anglo.

Variables: The sample is controlled by only one variable: the patient must be from one of the three cultures: Black-American, Spanish-American, or American Indian. Other controlled extraneous variables to be considered in the interaction include time of day; the culture, age, sex and status of the professional; the culture, sex, age and physical condition of the patient as well as his perception of his condition, his anxiety level and his diagnosis. These variables have been included in an *Observation Guide* for recording humorous interactions. It is recognized that there are other variables which cannot be controlled, but could be significant, such as the personality of both interactants and the degree of acculturation of the patient.

Data Collection:
1. Copies of *Observational Guides* which will be pretested and revised as needed will be provided each health professional who participates in the study.
2. Planned prediscussion periods with each group from an agency or unit will be conducted.

3. Two groups of recordings will be collected:
   a. Recalled humorous interactions from past experiences during the pre-discussion period.
   b. Those humorous interactions which occur in the following two weeks during their working hours.

The prediscussion period will be used to provide the health professionals with some background information on the concept of humor, the purpose of the study, and instructions on the use of the *Observation Guide*. During the discussion the health professionals will be encouraged to ask questions and express preconceived ideas in order to clear up misconceptions and to provide a mutual base for the observers.

Asking the professionals to recall past humorous interactions and record them on the *Observation Guide* should serve several purposes for the study:

1. To orient to the collection of data.
2. To give practice in using the *Guide*.
3. To stimulate interest in the study.
4. To increase the sample of humorous interactions.

Past experience with groups of persons during discussions about humor has resulted in an outpouring of remembered incidents. Asking busy people to collect and record data is not very productive unless they are stimulated to do so. The short time span for collection of data is also related to the fact that after the initial spurt of interest, the commitment fades and the material collected is not significant.

VI. Observation Guide

The *Observation Guide* is a modification of an initial one developed by the investigator in her first study, a further modification by Meechan in her graduate research project and subsequent revision during the present pretesting period. A written explanation for the use of the *Observation Guide* will be provided each observer.

REFERENCES

1. Coser RL: Some social functions of laughter: a study of humor in a hospital setting. *Human Relations* 12(2):171-182, 1959.
2. Fox RC: *Experiment Perilous.* Glencoe, Ill.: The Free Press, A. Corporation, 1959.
3. Emerson J: Social functions of humor in a hospital setting. Unpublished dissertation, University of California, 1963.
4. Robinson VM: Humor in nursing. *Behavioral Concepts and Nursing Intervention.* Coordinator, Carolyn Carlson. Philadelphia: JB Lippincott Company, 1970. 129-151.
5. Meechan PA: Humor use in patient-nurse interactions. Unpublished paper, University of Colorado, 1973.

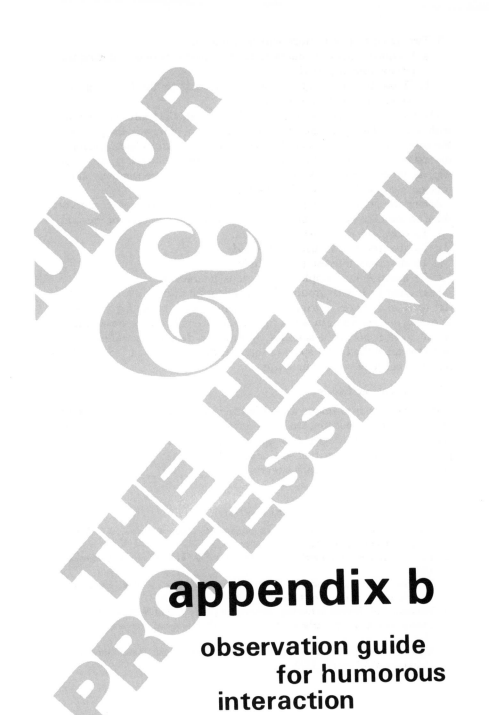

appendix b

observation guide
for humorous
interaction

Code _____   Name of Recorder: _____

OBSERVATION GUIDE FOR HUMOROUS INTERACTION

Setting: _____

Time of Day: Morning _____   Evening _____

Afternoon _____   Night _____

Information Re: Professional

Culture	Sex	Age	Profession
Anglo _____	Male _____	18-30 ____	R.N. _____
Black _____	Female _____	31-40 ____	LPN _____
Chicano _____		41-50 ____	Aide _____
Indian _____		51-60 ____	Other _____
		Over 60 ____	

Information Re: Patient

Culture	Sex	Age	Conditions
Black _____	Male _____	Under 6 ____	Acute _____
Chicano _____	Female _____	6-12 ____	Chronic _____
Indian _____		13-20 ____	Well _____
		21-30 ____	Convalescent _____
		31-40 ____	Satisfactory _____
		41-50 ____	Serious _____
		51-60 ____	Terminal _____
		Over 60 ____	

Patient's Perception of Condition:

Insignificant _____

Mildly serious _____

Moderately serious _____

Very serious _____

Terminal _____

Patient Appeared:

Relaxed _____

Mildly anxious _____

Moderately anxious _____

Very anxious _____

Denying seriousness _____

(continued on reverse side)

205

Diagnosis: _____
       (Nonobservational data)

State the situation in which the humor occurred: _____

_____

_____

Verbatim narrative of the humorous interaction: _____

_____

_____

_____

Result of Interaction:

Feeling Tone:

      Amusement _____
      Warmth _____
      Elation _____
      Flatness _____
      Anger _____
      Disgust _____
      Embarrassment _____

      Relief of tension _____
        Lessened anxiety _____
        Increased anxiety _____
      Led to expression of feelings _____
      Hindered expression of feelings _____
      Increased use of humor _____
      Facilitated relationship _____
      Hindered relationship _____

Other comments or observations: _____

_____

_____

_____

explanation of the observation guide for humorous interaction

Purpose:

The purpose of this guide is to record humorous incidents which occurred with patients from three different cultures: Black, Spanish-American, and American-Indian. These interactions may be those in which you participated or those which you observed occurring between another professional and a patient. The purpose of this investigation is to develop some beginning knowledge about the use of humor by members of the three cultures in times of stress such as illness and the reactions of those patients to the initiation of humor by health professionals.

Definition of Humor:

Humor is any communication which is perceived as humorous by any of the interacting parties and leads to laughing, smiling, or a feeling of amusement. This may be teasing, joking, witticisms, puns, clowning, joke-telling, a practical joke, a spontaneous funny which arose out of the interaction, etc.

Guide Details:

Setting: *e.g.,* hospital, medical ward, outpatient, emergency room, clinic, Center, home, etc.

Name of recorder: This provides the investigator the opportunity to contact the recorder if more information is needed.

Information Re: Patient and Professional:

These are the variables to be considered in the study which may be a consideration in the interaction.

**State the Situation in
which The Humor Occurred:**

This provides the framework in which the interaction took place: *i.e.,*
what activity was going on or what was the purpose of the contact (*e.g.,*
physical care, admission, interview, follow-up visit, etc.)

**Verbatim Narrative of
the Humorous Interaction:**

Record in your own words what occurred: (1) describe the interaction
leading up to the humor; and then (2) record verbatim conversation. The
exact words are important in conveying the humor rather than a
paraphrasing of it.

Result of Interaction:

Record your evaluation of the results of the humorous interaction, *e.g.,*
was there a pleasant positive feeling; did it fall flat; or was there a negative
reaction, a feeling of resentment or anger? Did the patient show relief or
lessened anxiety? Did it seem to facilitate your further interaction with the
patient? Did it help him to express his inner feelings or concerns or did it
lead to more humor? Negative reactions are as important to relate in your
evaluation as positive ones. Add any additional comments not outlined
that may be important observations.

INSTRUCTOR'S EVALUATION OF THE
GUIDE FOR THE USE OF HUMOR

1. Was it _____   _____ ? (Discuss)
        Useful   Not Useful

_____

_____

_____

_____

2. What was most useful? _____ .

3. What was least useful? _____ .

4. Did it give enough information? _____ .

5. Did it give too much detail? _____ .

6. Your suggestions for change, additions, deletions, etc.

_____

_____

7. Do you feel it has improved your ability to use humor? (Discuss)

_____

_____

_____

_____

INSTRUCTOR'S LOG

(To Accompany the Guide for the Use of
Humor in the Classroom)

Keep a running log of the humor used and include:

Course: _____ .

Subject matter: _____ .

Description of the humor or sample: _____

_____

_____ .

Reaction: (students and yours) _____

_____

_____ .

Any other comments, thoughts, etc. _____

_____

_____

_____

_____

_____ .

_____

_____

_____

STUDENT EVALUATION

Based upon the premise that humor facilitates learning, your instructor has been attempting to incorporate humor into his teaching. Would you evaluate his effort?

1. Did you notice? _____ .

2. What was the funniest bit of humor you remember? _____

_____

_____ .

3. Has it improved his teaching delivery? _____ .

4. Has it made the class more interesting? _____ .

5. Has it increased your learning? _____ .

6. Give examples of specific instances if you feel it has.

_____

_____

_____

_____ .

7. Other comments: _____

_____

_____

_____ .

_____